ALCOHOL AND THE DIET

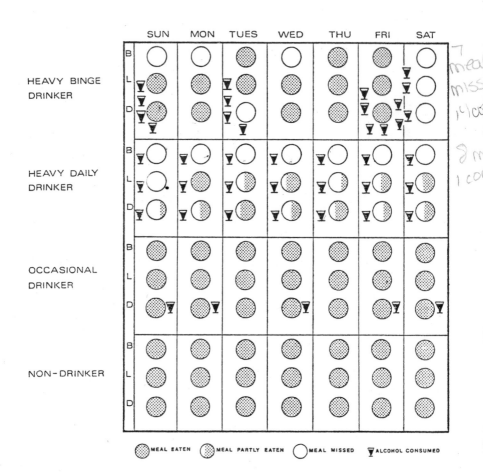

	SUN	MON	TUES	WED	THU	FRI	SAT
HEAVY BINGE DRINKER							
HEAVY DAILY DRINKER							
OCCASIONAL DRINKER							
NON-DRINKER							

⬡ MEAL EATEN   ⬡ MEAL PARTLY EATEN   ○ MEAL MISSED   ⴵ ALCOHOL CONSUMED

ALCOHOL AND THE DIET

Daphne A. Roe, M.D.

Professor of Nutrition
Cornell University
Ithaca, New York

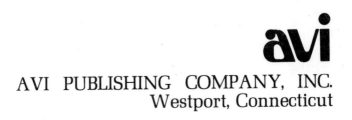

AVI PUBLISHING COMPANY, INC.
Westport, Connecticut

Library of Congress Cataloging in Publication Data ✓FDU Cat.

Roe, Daphne A
  Alcohol and the diet.

  ~~Includes index.~~
  ✓1. Alcoholism—Treatment—Nutritional aspects.
I. Title.
RC565.R553   616.8'61   79-214
✓ISBN O-87055-316-X

Printed in the United States of America

MLC

/A/311

Preface

The focus of this book is on the effects of alcoholic beverages and the diet on alcoholism with special emphasis on alcohol-nutrient interrelationships. After an introductory account of the folklore, convictions and the acquisitions of scientific information on alcohol and the diet, I have reviewed the effects of alcohol or alcohol abuse on nutritional status in such a way that consequences of drinking on eating habits, food intake, nutrient absorption and metabolism are described. The secondary effects of alcoholices on nutritional status are considered. Fetal malnutrition induced by alcohol is discussed. Nutritional assessment of alcoholics is described, following the guidelines now set for comprehensive determination of the nutritional status of patients in clinical settings. The chapter on nutritional rehabilitation of alcoholics has deliberately not been confined to an account of standard methods, but also contains suggestions for use of food behavior modification in treatment of alcoholics. Finally, I have included a short account of principal nutrient and non-nutrient components of alcoholic beverages and of drug-alcohol-food interactions.

While alcohol has long been recognized as a potent toxin, it is only within the last ten years that it has become generally accepted that most alcohol related diseases are the direct outcome of alcohol-induced tissue damage. Since both reversible and irreversible pathology can be attributed to alcohol abuse and not primarily to the defective diets consumed by alcoholics, the nutritional hazards of alcoholism have lately received less attention. However, currently, as in the past, the diets of alcoholics are commonly such as to place them at nutritional risk. Moreover, alcoholic damage to organs and tissues impairs nutrient absorption and utilization so that requirements for both macro and micronutrients are significantly altered.

Intended for all who are charged with the care of alcoholics, this book is particularly written for nutritionists, physicians, nurses, and phar-

macists who, in improving the quality of total patient care, must be concerned with the causes of alcoholic malnutrition, recognition of various
forms of malnutrition in their patients, and the importance of nutritional intervention in alcoholic patient management.

Readers should be dispelled of any notion that I have moral anti-
pathy to the fruit of the vine. I believe that undoubtedly, alcoholic
beverages contribute to the sensory appeal of food and the pleasurable
quality of many social occasions. However, we are a self-abusing
society, much given to excess in food as well as alcoholic consumption.
With respect to adverse effects on health, both habits are dangerous. As
Alexander Pope humorously cautioned his friends long ago,

> " 'T is yet in vain, I own, to keep up other
> About one vice, and fall into the other:
> Between Excess and Famine lies a mean"

(Alexander Pope. The Second Satire of the Second Book of Horace. To
Mr. Bethel. 1733-38.)

It is not my responsibility to offer a nutritional panacea for alcoholism, nor is there a magic diet for alcoholics. Readers must rest content
with the knowledge that I accept the fact that the conquest of alcoholism is not yet. The role of those who care for alcoholics is to improve
the quality of the patients' lives, to prevent nutritional diseases, and
perhaps to increase the functioning level of those who are or have been
alcohol-dependent. For those who accept these commitments, this book
is humbly dedicated.

Daphne A. Roe
Ithaca, N.Y.

February 26, 1979

Contents

Acknowledgements

I would like to thank my husband, Professor Albert Roe, for stimulating my research in the history of alcohol use, and for his unfailing encouragement to me as I wrote this book. I would also like to express my appreciation to the staff and research team of the Cornell Health Rehabilitation Project, who collected information on the diets and nutritional status of our alcoholic patients. I thank Mrs. Marion Van Soest for making the illustrations from my sketches. Finally, I owe a special debt of gratitude to Mrs. Beverly Hastings for her patient secretarial assistance in preparing the manuscript.

The author also wishes to express her appreciation to Dr. Norman W. Desrosier, Mrs. Shirley DeLuca and the AVI Publishing Company for encouragement and assistances in bringing this book into being.

The frontispiece, figures and values cited from other publications are reproduced with permission from museums, authors, and publishers.

Historical Accounts of Alcohol Use

FEASTING AND DRINKING IN ANCIENT TIMES

History suggests the obvious, that the use of alcohol parallels the availability of fermented liquors. Whereas the origin of the vine is in doubt, it was widely grown through the Middle East and the eastern Mediterranean area from about 3200 B.C. Darby *et al.* (1977) have given us a fascinating account of wine production in ancient Egypt and they allude to temple inscriptions mentioning joy from drinking as well as drunkenness. Wine was used by the Egyptians in religious celebrations, and also is listed among external applications and internal medications in the medical Papyri. Egyptian inscriptions, as well as tomb paintings, attest to the fact that drunkenness was associated with feasting, and that those who entertained the guests were more susceptible to intoxication, perhaps, than the guests themselves. Beer was also known from very early Egyptian times. It was considered as food and drink and in time became a popular beverage for the common people at times of festivity. As with wine, the Egyptians appreciated that if drunk to excess, beer caused inebriation.

Accounts of drunkenness in ancient Greece derived from Pliny, the Elder (Hist. Nat. XVI (28)). He alludes to the habitual drunkenness of guests at feasts and describes their behavior and appearance. Athenaeus (Athenaeus. III (C92)) mentions nations other than the Greeks including the Lydians, Persians, Scythians, Carthaginians, and Tapyri who were addicted to wine. The Macedonians were also drinkers and took large drafts of wine before meals to such an extent that they were unable to eat!

Rolleston (1927) found discussions of the gross excesses in drinking at Roman banquets in the works of Seneca (Seneca. XCV (95) C16). Romans at feasts had the habit of eating and drinking until they could take no more, and then vomiting was induced by tickling the throat with a flamingo or other bird's feather to reduce fullness so that further food and wine could be consumed. Inebriety was largely a matter of acute intoxication for the Greeks and Romans. Summarizing the characteristics of alcohol abuse among the ancients, Rolleston (1927) notes predominant incidence among the upper classes, lack of legislative control and an absence of distilled liquors.

In medieval times, drunkenness was prevalent, particularly among the lower orders of clergy who, at least in England, were said to have encouraged such excesses in their parishioners. We learn from Rolleston (1933a) that the Anglo-Saxons as well as their descendents drank ale, mead (wine and honey), morat (honey, mulberries and cider), and piment or pigment, the latter being a mixture of sour wine, honey and spices. In medieval England, wine was made from English grapes but wine was not plentiful until the end of the 14th century, when it was imported from France. There are descriptions of the acute effects of drinking in English medieval poetry. The following couplet, taken from Gower in his Confessio Amantis (1390) suggests a knowledge that drinking on an empty stomach is the quickest way to get drunk.

> He drynkth the wine but ate last
> The wine drynkth him and bint him faste.

Undoubtedly, ancient tradition provided medieval writers with prescriptions for the avoidance of drunkenness and its objectionable side effects. In pre-Norman British documents, we read that the best way to avoid loss of appetite which follows heavy drinking is to abstain (Cockayne, 1864-1866). The most expert English surgeon and scholar, John Arderne (1307-1390), proffers interesting dietary prescriptions against drunkenness, including the following mixture: juice of cabbage, 1 pint; juice of pomegranate, 1 pint; vinegar, half a measure; boil to ebullition and let an ounce be taken before drinking wine (Cockayne, 1864-1866). Darby et al. (1977) indicate that boiled cabbage was served at feasts when a lot of wine was going to be drunk during Egyptian times and that the tradition that cabbage could prevent drunkenness then persisted (Arderne, 1422).

Medieval aversion cures for habitual drunkenness give instructions for putting fish such as mullet into the wine, or alternatively, the lungs of a wild boar, or frogs should be similarly immersed, and the draft administered. The drunkard could otherwise take asses' or sows' milk in which an oyster or frog had been drowned (Rolleston, 1941).

ARDENT SPIRITS AND THE GIN EPIDEMIC

There is a tradition that from early times until the end of the medieval period episodic drinking and drunkenness were largely associated with revelry, feasting and religious celebration. Presumably, occupational alcoholism also has a very old tradition. The peasant laborer, working on the vines, might become an alcoholic since he drank wine he brought with him instead of water to relieve his thirst. Jellinek (1942) described the tradition of continuous imbibing in viti-cultural communities, and it is likely that associated alcoholism is as old as the culture of the grape. At least before the discovery of distillation, chronic alcoholism tended to be a personal or occupational problem which did not cause major social repercussions, nor the devastation of health of communities.

Alcoholism as a social problem really began with the production and availability of distilled beverages. It is known that primitive stills were adapted for the distillation of alcohol about 1100 A.D. (Singer, 1956). Aylward (1972) has stated that "This discovery led to the production of a wide variety of distilled spirits to supplement the older fermented beverages; it led also the production of a third group of beverages, namely wines or similar products fortified by the addition of alcohol." From the time of the discovery of distillation until the 16th century, production of liquors from wines was confined to monasteries and the production of fortified wines was on a relatively modest scale.

Lucia (1963), who has given us a very full account of the history of the discovery and use of fermented beverages and the distillation of alcohol, comments that the best evidence suggests that Franciscus Sylvius (or Franz de la Boe), a 17th century professor of medicine at the University of Leiden, may have been the first to distill alcohol from grain. Sylvius called this new alcoholic beverage "Aqua Vitae." In Holland, this drink was known as "Junever," which is the Dutch word for juniper, the berry with which the alcohol was usually flavored, to mask the taste of the crude spirit. The French used the term "Genièvre." The English translated Genièvre to Geneva, and then shortened this word to Gin.

Gin, or "Holland's," was produced in the Netherlands in the 17th century and was imported into England during the reign of William III. H.B. Wheatley alludes to a tradition that it was the King himself who first brought in this beverage from his native country (Wheatley, 1909). Lord Kinross (1959) considers that some gin was brought to England earlier by soldiers returning from the wars in the Netherlands in the early 17th century. The soldiers were convinced that the gin gave them "Dutch courage." Importation and distribution of the gin was very limited at that time, because of favorable economics policies toward the bringing in to England of wines and brandies from the Continent. Whether or not William III actually brought gin to England, or increased its importation, more Dutch gin was brought into England during the latter part of the 17th century. However, by 1700, production of distilled liquors, mainly gin, in England was also a profitable industry. The ill effects of drinking this form of ardent spirits did not long go unnoticed. Whereas in 1690 the British government passed legislation to support distillation, in 1695 Charles Davenant pointed out the health risks of both gin and brandy: "And if as physicians sayeth (strong waters) extinguishes natural heat and apetite, it hinders the consumption of Flesh and corn in a degree. Tis a growing vice among the common people...." He recommended that a tax be imposed on liquor which would make it inaccessible to the poor but his advice fell on deaf ears.

Dorothy George (1931) notes that "distilling had been encouraged by the government as a remedy for the over-production of corn, which was then thought to be a danger to the whole agricultural interest." According to Hirsch (1949), the English distilling industry was given impetus through animosity to France and prejudice against French products. English gin and whiskey manufacture were therefore supported and high tariffs were imposed on French wine. In any case, according to Lucia (1963), the public response to the British government's legislation of 1690, "An act for the encouraging of the distillation of brandy and spirits from corn," was most enthusiastic.

Early in the 18th century, freedom was granted in England to anyone to distill liquor if notice was first given to the Commissioner of Excise, and if they were willing to pay the low excise duty then required. Retailing of gin and other spiritous liquors could be carried out without the special Justice's License, which was demanded from ale-house keepers. Dorothy George (1925), who extracted this information from contemporary documents, emphasizes that following the freedoms granted to the distilling trade, two types of distillers made their appearance. These were the malt distillers, who produced raw spirits, and were few in number, and the compound distillers, or rectifiers, who concocted a variety of gin drinks which they flavored variously with juniper berries, and anise seeds, as well as adulterants. The cheap gin sold to the masses in London was potent and toxic.

Examination of the gin drinking epidemic which followed the first excessive liquor production in England affords us the opportunity to see the social effects of alcohol abuse when liquor availability was entirely uncontrolled. The high death rate and low birth rate within the London area that is recorded in Bills of Mortality between 1720-1750 are explained by Dorothy George as being a consequence of alcoholism, particularly among the poor. A campaign against the drinking of gin and brandy began about 1721, but in the years that followed was remarkably unsuccessful at bringing about restrictive government action. There was a great proliferation in the retailers of gin, and it was sold not only from shops such as chandlers, but also from stalls, back rooms and even wheelbarrows. Contemporary observers, having social insight, noted the inverse relationship between gin consumption and socioeconomic status. The poor were attracted to gin drinking primarily by its availability and its cheapness, which compared favorably with the cost of other beverages, and by its ability to ameliorate hunger, misery and a squalid environment. By social analogy, we can compare the gin drinking epidemic of the early to mid-18th century with the determinants of heroin addiction in the 1960's.

Prohibition of gin retailing in 1736 by Parliamentary edict was a complete failure. Opposing viewpoints were indicated by the comment of a pamphleteer writing in the year 1736: "The distillers are the farmers' great friends . . . what would become of our corn injured by bad harvest were it not for the distillers?" (Allen, 1736).

An anonymous engraving, made in 1736 and presently in the possession of the British Museum, is entitled "The Funeral Procession of Madam Geneva." The superscript reads "To those Melancholly Sufferers (by a severe act) the Distillers, this plate is most humbly Inscrib'd by a lover of Trade." The design shows a street with a spirits shop on one side; over the door is written: "Geneva, Brandy, Rum, Arrack, Ca-." A funeral procession approaches the burial ground and a nearly naked beggar follows the coffin as chief mourner. There is also a long procession of publicans dressed in black. On the coffin is a dram glass, a measure for spirits, and a small keg. In the foreground are women drinking and fighting and showing effects of drunkenness. The subscript consists in a poem ending with lines which indicate an awareness that indigent people were most likely to drink gin:

> How vast those patriots publick Spirit
> To strip the poor of their chief Pleasure
> And Thousands leave to starve at Leasure.

(Catalog of Prints and Drawings of the British Museum, 1934). Apparently as the time (the 29th of September, 1736) approached when the "Act of Suppressing Geneva" was to come into effect, retail dealers in gin put their shop signs in mourning and made a mock funeral parade for Madam Geneva.

The first half of the 18th century and particularly the years from 1720-1750 in England are not only marked by an unprecedented wave of alcohol consumption by lower income people, but also this was the period when the adverse nutritional and health effects of alcoholism were first recognized. However, recognition of these effects took second place to public concern over the social consequences of alcohol consumption. One of the most outspoken writers against the social corruption, moral degradation, and health devastation of alcoholism, was Henry Fielding. In 1751, at the time when he had just become a magistrate, his book "*An Enquiry into the Causes of the Late Increase of Robbers, etc.*" was published. The second section of this book, entitled "*Of Drunkenness*," comprises a discussion of the consequences of "luxury among the vulgar." Luxury, in this sense, suggests improper use of leisure time. Fielding herein refers to a tract entitled "*Distilled Spiritous Liquors, The Bane of the Nation*"—composed by a very learned Divine with the assistance of several physicians and published in the year 1736. Zirker (1966) has proven that Fielding's information concerning the devastating social and health effects of gin were obtained from this tract by the "Very Learned Divine," a certain Thomas Wilson (1703-1784), who expressed his views in these words: "The Greatest Part of the Nation, that Part which is the Strength and Riches of every country, the Laborious Hands, is intoxicated and enervated by a fatal Love of a slow but sure Poyson, which enters into the Blood and Marrow of its Habitual Drinkers and transmits its deadly Effects into the vitals of their miserable Posterity..." (Wilson, 1736).

Fielding's knowledge of the effects of alcoholism was clearly much influenced by this writing, which, as he recounts, gives "the physical account of the nature of all distilled spiritous liquors and the effects they have on human bodies." Fielding refers to "a new kind of drunkenness which will infallably destroy a great part of our inferior people..." "What," he exclaims, "must become of the infant who is conceived in gin?...Doth not this polluted source promise only to fill alms houses and hospitals and to infect the street with stench and diseases?"

A few weeks after the appearance of Fielding's Enquiry, Hogarth's famous prints "Gin Lane" and "Beer Street" were published. "Gin Lane" is a strong, graphic expression of Fielding's account of a pitiable state of the gin drinking poor (Figure 1:1). Antal (1952) writes, "Hogarth's Gin Lane and Beer Street, also published in 1751 . . . were designed to give strong support to the latter's arguments placing drunkenness, particularly excessive gin drinking, as among the main

GIN LANE

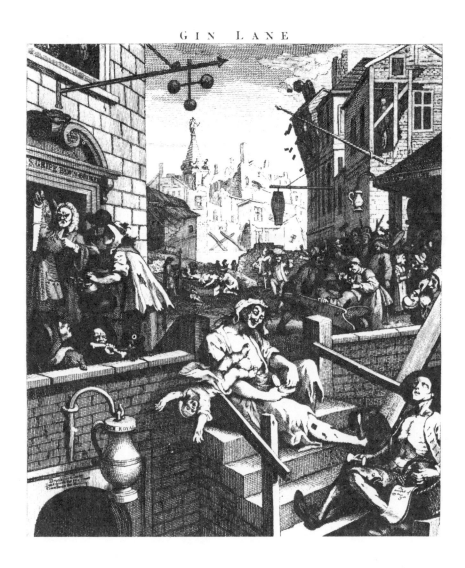

FIG. 1.1. GIN LANE. FROM HOGARTH'S GRAPHIC WORKS, 1751.

causes not only of criminality, idleness and immorality, but also of the undermining of health." In Antal's paper, attention is drawn on the one hand to the fact that to Hogarth, beer drinking was considered to be associated with virtue, whereas gin drinking was associated with vice. The impact of Hogarth's "Gin Lane" has been attributed by Coffey (1966) to the wide distribution of the print, which was sold for a shilling. He intimates that, since the public's conscience had been aroused by the pictorial demonstration of the consequences of gin drinking, the government had to take action, despite opposition from vested interests.

Both Fielding's Enquiry and Hogarth's Gin Lane were used effectively to bring pressure on the government to institute legislation against the production and sales of gin. Petitions from various sources including the Corporation of London, from London parishes as well as from several other cities to the House of Commons were received during 1751. These petitions pointed out the lethal effects of cheap liquor, as well as the relationship between drunkenness and idleness or disordered behavior (Dorothy George, 1925).

Verses which appeared in the *General Advertisor* for March 7, 1751 indicate that malnutrition secondary to alcohol excesses were being brought to the public notice:

> *Strip-Me-Naked, Or Royal Gin Forever*
> "I must, I will have gin! - that skillet take:-
> Pawn it:-no more our roast, or boil or bake.
> This Juice immortal will each Want supply,
> Starve on (ye brats)! So I but bung my Eye.
> Starve? No!-This Gin doth Mother's Milk excell;
> Will paint the Cheeks and Hunger's Darts Repell.-"

The Gin Act was passed in 1751 (24 Geo. II c. 40). It imposed a duty on spirits and stopped distillers, chandlers and grocers from retailing liquor. The Webbs (1903) have indicated that the Gin Act was followed by a marked reduction in the sale of spirits. However, we should not construe this to mean that the epidemic of gin drinking was promptly curtailed. Indeed, many years elapsed before this first epidemic of alcohol excess was brought under control.

SOCIAL CAUSES AND CONSEQUENCES OF HABITUAL DRUNKENNESS

Caution should be exercised in considering that in the 18th century gin was the only liquor leading to alcoholism in a large social group. The English episode of alcoholism was a prototype based on gin. The 18th century was a time of widespread alcoholic excess among different strata of society, both in Europe and in the American Colonies. The well-to-do indulged in wine and brandy, but did not have to make the choice between eating or drinking. Assisted by their friends and families, well endowed alcoholics were able to support their habit, and may have avoided some of the alcoholic diseases through abundant food intake. The autobiographical detail provided by James Boswell, friend of Dr. Johnson, gives a remarkable picture of the life and times of an educated alcoholic in the latter half of the 18th century (Rix, 1975). Despite blackouts and periods of forgetfulness, he was socially accepted.

In the 18th century, as in later times, the poor and those subservient to others, bore the burden of the combined effects of alcoholism and social misery. Alcoholism became prevalent in certain occupational groups in the late 17th and 18th centuries because of deliberate encouragement of drinking in order that men might perform unpleasant or highly dangerous tasks. There was also a belief that drinking, even hard drinking, was an attribute of manliness. Similarly, a tradition of alcohol abuse was fostered in sailors and soldiers, because beer or liquor might increase endurance or add to physical strength.

Rum was first produced in 1650, being developed in the Caribbean as a by-product of the sugar cane industry, which was supported by slave labor. The first rum was distributed to men in the Royal Navy in 1692, and this liquor contained 80% of alcohol by volume. Admiral Vernon, a contemporary supporter of rum for sailors, suggested that the rum would be more palatable and safer if diluted with water. He believed that a rum ration not only conferred strength, but also gave protection against scurvy (Chalke, 1976). The diarist, Pepys, however, at a slightly earlier date, recognized the prevalence of alcoholism in the Royal Navy (Rolleston, 1944). Undoubtedly the sailors of those days had access to other liquor when in port, but as French, in 1891 has suggested, alcoholism among sailors may have been fostered by the distribution of rum grog.

Further insights into the risks of drink for the 18th century sailor can best be judged by reading Blane's *Observations on the Diseases of Seamen* (1785). Dr. Blane, who had been a physician to the British Fleet, describes the diet of the sailors as consisting mainly of salted meats with some bread and biscuit. At sea, virtually no vegetables were provided, other than occasional "sourkrout." Oranges and lemons or cordials made from these fruits were largely kept for men with advanced scurvy. We are told by Blane that the sailors very frequently developed sores that would not heal, and this evidence suggests that they were, in fact, scorbutic. Other deficiency diseases, including vitamin A deficiency, are suggested by Blane's narrative, which alludes to nightblindness. Blane comments, "When a ship is in port, encouragement should be given to the sale of roots, greens, fruits, and sugar. The men have a good custom of exchanging part of their bread, beef and pork for what they can get from the shore, but as they prefer spiritous liquor to the above mentioned articles, the greatest care and vigilance should be used to preclude men from such opportunities of injuring themselves."

Puritans in the American Colonies believed that alcoholic drinks were wholesome and that drinking such beverages could help them to withstand the rigors to which they were exposed. Beer was considered as a form of sustenance. In the early days of the Colonies, distilled spirits were not available, which was perhaps a fortunate situation. When, in the 18th century, rum and whiskey were either imported, or in the case of whiskey, locally produced, the upright colonists came rapidly to realize the potential dangers of alcohol abuse. Black slaves and American Indians were considered too irresponsible to be trusted with the use of alcohol, and it was indeed a punishable offense to provide alcohol to slaves. Nevertheless, the less scrupulous colonists paid no attention to this law, and very quickly spiritous liquors were used to appease the Indians and as a sop to the slaves to perform unpleasant duties (Bourne, 1973).

In a tract published in 1774 without recognizable authorship, but by "a lover of mankind," we can read of the tragic consequences of the illicit use and abuse of alcohol by Blacks and Indians (Benezet, 1774). According to this author, who quotes figures from the *Pennsylvania Gazette*, a total of 224,500 gallons of rum were imported into this Colony alone in one year (1728), which he intimates, may have become available for the Indian trade. We assume that more rum followed for consumption by the Indians. Anyway, in 1753, the chief of the Six Nations convened a meeting in which he expressed horror that the Colonies' promise of trade had turned out to be a trade in whiskey and rum, and he begged that this might be stopped. Elsewhere in this publication, it is remarked that "the destructive effect of distilled spirits have also extended their bainful influence through the peoples of Africa." We may assume that the evil influence of the liquor may have been malnutrition. This anonymous American author's maxims are of special interest: "Nothing," he writes, "conduces more to health and long life than abstinence and plain food with due labor. Water alone is sufficient and effective for all the purposes of human want to drink. It is the universal dissolvant nature has provided, and the most certain diluter of all bodies proper for food, quickens the appetite and strengthens digestion . . . strong and spiritous liquors were never designed for common use. They were formerly kept in England as other medicines are in apothecary shops . . . The great quantity of viscid malt liquor drunk by the common people of England cannot fail to render the blood fizy."

ALCOHOL-INDUCED DISEASES AND ALCOHOLISM

Reasonably accurate accounts of the health problems of alcoholics can be found in medical literature from the early years of the 18th century, and what is interesting to us is that there are many instances where 18th century and early 19th century authors appear to understand relationships between alcohol abuse and nutritional disorders. Sedgwick in 1725 described the results of "the attackment of drunkenness" in the following words: "The reasons why it is followed by so many diseases is because in a drunken condition, a vast quantity of blood is thrown into the brain and those parts nearest to the heart whereby the tone of their fiber is destroyed (especially if drunkenness is often repeated) and they become so weak as not to be able to carry out the circulation of the humours. For which reason hard drinkers will be stupid and subject to apoplexies, palsies, vertigo, loss of memory, trembling of the hands, a bad digestion, tumours of the liver, spleen or mesentery from whence proceed a jaundice and dropsy, the common fate of most great drinkers." The author acknowledges his indebtedness to Sir John Floyer and a certain Dr. Wainwright for source material on the effects of alcohol, but does not give recognizable references. He also shows a rather excessive concern for the ill effects of water, which no doubt was the source of infection in his day.

John Coakley Lettsom (1792), a gifted Quaker physician, biologist and social reformer, had outstanding powers of observing the human condition. He was perhaps the first to consider alcoholism per se as a disease. In 1786, he read a paper before the Medical Society of London, later published in the Proceedings of that Society. In a description of the treatment of dyspepsia, in people who have indulged in hard drinking, he intimates that he is aware that alcoholism occurs in women as well as in men, and that he knows that it is more likely to develop in those whose situations in life have undergone a change (Fig. 1.2).He also describes anorexia, pyloric stenosis secondary to peptic ulcer, and pancreatitis in alcoholics (Rix, 1976).

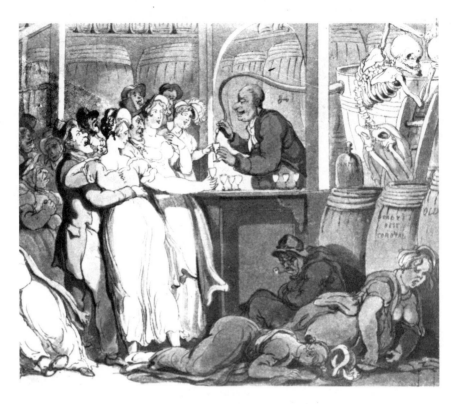

FIG. 1.2.   SOME FIND THEIR DEATH BY SWORD & BULLET; AND
SOME BY FLUIDS DOWN THE GULLET

Dr. Thomas Trotter (1804) was another early medical writer on alcoholism, and was the first to provide his students with a more complete catalog of alcohol-related disorders and diseases. He cites a list of conditions induced by repeated drunkenness in a little book first published in 1802. These include apoplexy, epilepsy, hysteria, fearful dreams, madness, melancholy, inflammatory disease of the liver, gout, schirrus (hardening disease of the bowels), jaundice, dyspepsia, dropsy, emaciation, impotency, diabetes, premature old age, and in children, breast-fed by alcoholic wet nurses, dullness, drowsiness, and stupidity. Discussing the anorexia of alcoholism, he writes, "even when some appetite remains, the food gives no support"—an excellent description of alcoholic cachexia.

The use of ardent spirits in the United States was chiefly the result of the availability of cheap rum. Dr. Benjamin Rush, writing in 1809, observed: "It is highly probable not less than 4,000 people die annually from the use of ardent spirits in the United States. Should they continue to exert this deadly influence upon our population, where will their evils terminate?... They have perished, not by pestilence nor war, but by a greater foe to human life than either of them... ardent spirits... To avert this evil let good men of every class unite and beseech the general and state governments with petitions to limit the number of taverns; to impose heavy duties upon ardent spirits; to inflict a mark of disgrace, or a temporary abridgement of some civil right upon every man convicted of drunkenness; and finally to secure the property of habitual drunkards for the benefit of their families, by placing it in the hands of trustees appointed for that purpose by a court of justice." (See Table 1.1).

TABLE 1.1   FEDERAL EXCISE TAX RATES ON DISTILLED SPIRITS

Year	Rate[1] ($)	Year	Rate[1] ($)
1791 (July)	0.09-0.25	1894 (Aug.)	1.10
1792 (July)	0.07-0.15	World War I	2.30
1802 (July)	No tax	1919 (Febr.)	6.40
1815 (Jan.)	0.09	1933 (Dec.)	1.10
1818 (Jan.)	No tax	1934 (Jan.)	2.00
1862 (Sept.)	0.20	1938 (July)	2.25
1864 (March)	0.60	1940 (July)	3.00
1864 (July)	1.50	1941 (Oct.)	4.00
1864 (Dec.)	2.00	1942 (Nov.)	6.00
1868 (July)	0.50	1944 (April)	9.00
1872 (Aug.)	0.70	1951 (Nov.)	10.50
1875 (March)	0.90	currently	10.50

[1]Per tax gallon.
Source: Packowski (1974)

Rush had a good knowledge, insight and experience of the effects of hard drinking and chronic alcoholism. He describes loss of appetite, "sickness at stomach," "obstructions of the liver," jaundice, dropsy, diabetes, redness of the face (rum-buds or rosacea), fetid breath, epilepsy, gout and madness. It is of interest to us that Rush distinguishes the kind of anorexia found after an acute drinking bout, which is of short duration, from anorexia due to chronic alcoholism which is most severe in the morning and which is associated with disease of the gastrointestinal system. Rush does not discuss the changes in the accustomed food intake of alcoholics, but he does make the statement: "A diet consisting wholly of vegetables cured a physician in Maryland of drunkenness, probably by lessening that thirst which is always more or less excited by animal food." Although Rush correctly associated specific health problems with alcoholism, and particularly emphasized disease of the liver as a complication, he could also believe the folklore about drunkards which was extant in his time.

For example, he follows the statement that "frequent and disgusting belchings" are symptoms of chronic drinking by relating a case described by a certain Doctor Haller of a well-known drunkard who died after a vaporous discharge from his stomach caught fire following contact with a candle flame!

In his writings on alcoholism and alcoholics, Rush was much influenced by his contemporaries and by earlier authors. Indeed, his renown relates more to his missionary zeal to prevent or treat alcoholism than to his recorded observations (Rush, 1943).

Perhaps because of overwhelming evidence since the early 18th century, of the reality of alcoholism as a social problem, it has been assumed that the modern concept of alcoholism has been accepted since that time. Bynum (1968) has cast doubt on this theory. He says, "The concept of chronic alcoholism as a disease instead of merely as a vice or a cause of other diseases developed only within modern times." He considers that medical interests in the harmful effects of drinking began about the turn of the 18th century, and that this was followed by a long period running into the 19th century, when alcohol was considered to be a cause of various diseases. Words like alcoholism or alcoholismus to express a dependence on alcohol, as well as the collective mental and physical effects of alcohol belong to the last century and to our own times. However, because the word alcoholism was not used until the 19th century does not mean that the diagnostic criteria were not understood either by self-diagnosed alcoholics or by those who observed them. Indeed, Bynum has explained that the term "habitual drunkenness" signified the physical state now described as chronic alcoholism. The artificial and erroneous fragmentation of diseases associated with alcohol, as well as the persistent preoccupation with the sinful nature of alcohol use and abuse, belong to Temperance literature where the lay or clerical writers were deliberately attempting to arouse public opinion against perceived evils of alcoholic drinks.

Brühl-Cramer in 1819 defined dipsomania as an abnormal craving for alcohol. What is interesting to us about this definition is that he made analogies with special food cravings, including, for example, in intermittent fever, a desire for exotic foods that are harmful and the envy of the pregnant woman. This is the first publication in which the predisposition of the alcoholic to drink is defined, and Brühl-Cramer's ideas herald the modern concept of alcoholism as an aberrant psychological state.

The toxic effects of alcohol on human tissues and organs which we now know can directly or indirectly cause nutritional disorders derive from the teachings of Fuchs and Magnus Huss. Fuchs (1845-1848) described alcohol as a poison, and classified alcoholism with other poisonings such as arsenical and mercurial intoxication and ergotism. Huss (1852) perceived that the effects of chronic alcohol abuse were to induce tissue damage. He further subscribed to the concept that the toxic effects of alcohol resemble in some aspects those induced by inappropriate foods. However, whereas he recognized that effects of alcohol on tissues outside the central nervous system were prejudicial to the health of alcoholics, his central theme of alcohol as a disease pertains to the mental and neurological effects. Bynum (1968) has recognized that Huss described the symptoms of Korsakoff's psychosis which is seen in alcoholics and of nutritional etiology, forty years before the man who gave his name to the syndrome (Korsakoff, 1889).

Historical accounts of associations between alcoholism and malnutrition belong to more recent times. Two concepts must be introduced. The first of these is that alcoholics, because they eat badly, may be particularly vulnerable for the development of nutritional diseases, as for example, vitamin deficiencies; and secondly, the tissue damage associated with alcoholism may be due to nutritional deficiency. Predating the modern science of nutrition and an appreciation of the role of individual nutrients for the maintenance of the economy of the body, are observations of the prevalence of diseases now known to be endemic nutritional diseases among alcohol addicts. From the historical standpoint, delay in the recognition that alcoholics are likely to suffer multiple nutritional deficiencies can be explained as a failure to understand dietary habits which would place alcoholics at high nutritional risk. Minot et al. (1933) noted that "Man seldom chooses his food so as to create a condition due to the deficiency of only one substance." If in this quotation we substitute an alcoholic for the word man, it is easy to appreciate why the alcoholics' nutritional deficiencies are somewhat difficult to recognize, since the deficiency of one nutrient may be superimposed upon the other because of the low levels of several nutrients in the diet. Failure to recognize nutritional deficiencies among alcoholics led to the development of terms such as "alcoholic" polyneuritis and "pseudo" pellagra. Jolliffe (1940) has commented on a rather widespread failure on the part of physicians and nutritionists to recognize that these diseases were in fact true vitamin deficiencies. He describes the role of alcohol in the development of nutritional deficiency disease, dividing causal relationships into four categories:

1. The association of gastrointestinal disturbances associated with excessive alcohol intake which result in dietary restriction.
2. Alcohol can produce changes in the gastrointestinal tract which

lead to an interference in the absorption and utilization of vitamins.

3. Alcohol may be substituted for vitamin-containing food.

4. There may be an increased vitamin requirement, secondary to the provision of calories as alcohol.

Jolliffe is the first to point out that "an individual consuming an adequate diet may, merely by the addition of alcohol calories, make the diet an inadequate one..." These statements are more or less in keeping with our present ideas on the interrelationships between alcohol intake and nutritional status. They should be compared, perhaps, with beliefs of a previous generation, just thirty years earlier, when it was considered that alcoholics, like the insane, were particularly vulnerable to develop certain diseases, presumably because of their bad blood. For example, Dr. James Babcock, a pioneer in mapping the incidence of pellagra in the United States is acknowledged by Tucker (1911) as the originator of the idea that alcoholics are prone to develop pellagra because they are particularly susceptible to the toxin elaborated by moldy corn.

ALCOHOL IN MEDICINE

Wines, beer, and later spirits have been used in the treatment of many kinds of disease. Indeed, alcoholic beverages were considered as the sovereign stimulant to rouse a patient's recuperative powers. As has been previously mentioned, belief in the healing power of wine derives from Egyptian times. Rolleston (1929) has also provided evidence for us that there is a tradition that Homer used wine as an application to wounds. In classical literature, wine is advocated as an ingredient of therapeutic diets by Plautus, Lucretius, Ovid, Juvenal and Martial.

So ingrained was the medical tradition of alcohol in therapeutics that it did not die out until about fifty years ago. Indeed, the reaction against the use of alcohol as a drug only began in the early 19th century and parallels the development of the Temperance movement. The early supporters of the movement first began to question the need for alcohol as a restorative of health and later supporters instituted clinical research with the objective of demonstrating that alcohol could be deleted from the pharmacopeia.

In tracing the decline of alcohol as a wonder drug, it is important to reflect that it was the development of the practice of dietetics which most influenced medical opinion. Until it was shown that food could positively influence recovery from acute and chronic disease, and that alcohol did not have this beneficial effect, prescription of wines and liquors continued.

Although it is intimated by the authors of Temperance literature that the ineffectiveness of alcohol as a therapeutic agent was appreciated by the medical profession, at least since the 18th century and perhaps much earlier, historical research indicates that the number of medical men in the 18th century even suggesting restraint in the use of alcohol in disease were very few. Winskill (1881) associates the medical profession with the early history of the Temperance movement. The number of physicians who were associated with the Temperance movement were relatively few. A forerunner of the Medical Temperance Brotherhood was John Higginbottom, surgeon, who Rolleston (1933b) discovered had experimentally discontinued the use of alcohol in the treatment of his patients in 1832.

Formulation of alcoholic drafts for the treatment of special diseases or the alleviation of certain symptoms was a most respectable medical exercise, particularly popular in the middle 19th century. Todd's Potion, a draft containing rum, was advocated for the treatment of fevers. This particular mixture was named after Dr. Bentley Todd, who lectured on the subject in 1860. Todd believed that alcohol was an antidote for erysipelas (Todd, 1860).

While being critical of alcoholic medications such as Todd's mixture, which consisted of rum and tincture of cinnamon in a syrup (Martindale, 1972), a fellow London physician, Dr. F.E. Anstie, had a widespread influence in supporting the need for wines in the control of both acute and chronic health problems. He particularly advised wine be given in conditions "due to greatly increased tissue waste...," and he suggested that wine, preferably Rhenish or Hungarian wine, or "splendid old sherry" were the supportive treatments of choice in bronchitis and pneumonia, as well as in "catarrhal diarrhea." In non-febrile disorders, Anstie cautions physicians against "routine alcoholisation," but then recommends wine for the treatment of hemorrhage, acute neuroses, chorea, acute neuralgia, shock and debility. In chlorosis or iron deficiency anemia, he explains that port should be given, and no other wine; whereas "steel wine" should be administered to children with rickets and a mixture of quinine and alcohol was Anstie's remedy for chronic infection (Anstie, 1877).

Pediatric literature in the middle and late 19th century abounds with favorable comments on the effects of alcohol on the outcome of children's diseases. Thus in a standard text by Dr. Eustace Smith (1884) we learn "Children reduced by severe illness respond well to the action of alcohol . . . Children with poor appetites and feeble digestions often benefit greatly from an allowance of wine with their principal meal." Choleraic summer diarrhea (probably a manifestation of protein-calorie malnutrition) was, according to this author, to be controlled by doses of brandy to be given every few minutes while chronic diarrhea would better respond to an egg and brandy mixture.

As recently as 1905, Robert Hutchison, a distinguished British physician, is still advocating liquor as a treatment for fevers, and he is very specific about the type of alcohol which should be administered. In giving advice to physicians and perhaps nurses, he writes: "The form in which alcohol should be given in fevers is not a matter of indifference. If one merely wishes to obtain its effects upon the temperature and circulation any pure form of spirit will do. Sound malt whiskey is as good as any other. Where, however, there are signs of nervous exhaustion—as, for example, in the 'typhoid state'—a preparation rich in volatile ethers should be selected. Of these, genuine cognac is one of the best, and it is worthwhile to pay a high price for it in order to be sure of having it good...In catarrhal conditions, and where a tendency to vomiting is present, an effervescing wine, such as good, dry, champagne, often gives the best result...In deciding upon the amount of alcohol to be given and the frequency of its administration one must be guided chiefly by the urgency of the indications calling for its use. Half an ounce of spirit diluted with twice as much water, or an ounce of one of the stronger wines may be given every 4, 3 or 2 hours according to the effect produced or even every hour if occasion demands it." (Hutchison, 1905).

Hutchison's remarks are particularly illustrative of the prevailing medical opinion in his time. As for example, "There are grounds also for the belief that alcohol actually increases the resisting power of the body to the poisons of certain diseases— . . . In some chronic diseases, such as diabetes, alcohol is used as a real food to replace a certain amount of carbohydrate in the diet, whilst in others it is chiefly its tonic influences on digestion which one often seeks to obtain." (Hutchison, 1905).

Sir Victor Horsley (1907) gave wholehearted support to the claims by scientists and laity associated with the Temperance movement, that alcohol lacks the properties of a nutrient. "Alcohol," he writes, "has never been shown to produce energy for muscular work." He further makes the statement, "Substances which are truly dietetic enter into the composition of the normal chemistry of the human organism (a property which cannot be claimed for alcohol)." He demolishes the arguments of his colleagues, who cannot believe that the sick can be managed without alcoholic stimulants. He notes that alcohol impairs rather than stimulates food intake; it does not aid digestion but may disguise dyspepsia, and that it has adverse effects on taste perception.

He refutes the then current belief that alcohol is a stomach dis-infectant. Discussing the administration of alcohol to women after childbirth, he emphasizes that this will make lactation deficient and contribute to infant mortality. In general, he finds no good evidence that alcohol aids in therapy, but rather that it has deleterious effects on the sick and convalescent patient.

Sir Victor showed both graphically and in table form that from 1865-1905 there was a reduction in the use of alcohol in hospitals, and that this decrease in alcohol consumption was associated directly with an increase in the consumption of milk by hospital patients (Fig. 1.3).

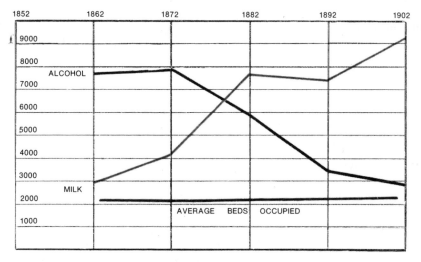

Diagram in continuation of Dr. Hare's Table showing the gradual diminution during the past forty years in the administration of Alcohol and the increase in the use of Milk during the same period. The figures are summarized from the statistics of seven large London Hospitals.

FIG. 1.3. HOSPITAL STATISTICS FOR ALCOHOL ADMINISTRATION AND MILK CONSUMPTION IN 7 LONDON HOSPITALS, 1862–1902 (HORSLEY AND STURGE, 1907).

However, vast quantities of wine, beer, and liquor were used in British hospitals, including the prestigous teaching hospitals of Lon-don throughout the 19th century. Rolleston (1928) has indicated that, whereas, there was some decline in expenditures per patient for wines, whiskey and brandy after about 1860 in teaching hospitals, even as recently as 1923 alcohol was very much in vogue for the treatment of acute infections by fever hospitals. He traces the persistent use of alcohol in acute disease to three factors: 1) tradition, 2) extra-medical influences, by which he means the opinions of the lay public, and 3) personal factors including ignorance by members of the medical profession that frequent administration of alcohol as a drug could lead to alcoholism.

In 1923, he conducted experiments at the London Fever Hospital, in which alternating patients admitted with typhus were either given repeated doses of 4-12 fluid ounces of brandy, or were put on a regime of milk and beef tea. The rate of recovery was similar in the two groups. However, in spite of these findings, alcohol was still used six years later at this hospital in the treatment of pneumonia, typhoid, diphtheria, and other infections. Interesting figures are given by Rolleston on the declining use of brandy in the Western Fever Hospital in the middle-1920's and associated changes in the diphtheria mortality (Table 1.2).

TABLE 1.2   TABLE INDICATING CONSUMPTION OF BRANDY AT WESTERN FEVER HOSPITAL

Quarters	1925	1926	1927
1st	798 oz.	914 ½ oz.	5 oz.
2nd	344	61 ½	12
3rd	340	13	5
4th	1107	2 ½	3 ½
Total	2589	991 ½	25 ½
Diptheria Mortality	8.54 percent	4.42 percent	3.01 percent

Ref: Rolleston, J.D. Alcohol in acute infectious diseases.
   Brit. J. Inebriety 25: 201-203, 1928.

ALCOHOL AS FOOD

By ancient tradition, wine and beer were considered as food, acceptable by the sick when solid food could not be tolerated. When spirits became available they, too, were accepted by the medical profession and the laity as appropriate nourishment both for debilitated persons and for those who refused to eat in times of sickness. It was the Temperance workers of the 19th century who encouraged and supported studies to determine the food value of alcohol. The first experiments of any note were those by Lallemand, Perrin and Duroy in 1860, who made several studies using men and dogs. The doses of alcohol administered were generally large, and in some cases when the alcohol was given to the dogs, the dogs died. They found that some alcohol was given off from the body unoxidized, and since no large amounts of alcohol metabolites were isolated from tissue or excreta, they inferred that the greater part of the alcohol was eliminated unchanged. Experiments conducted between 1865 and 1874 by Anstie (1864, 1874), Thudichum (1868), and Dupré (1871, 1872) formed the basis of the opposite conclusion, that alcohol as ordinarily taken, is nearly completely oxidized in the body.

Atwater *et al.* (1900, 1903) have given us an extensive account of these investigations and of others intended to define whether alcohol can be considered as a food. In these discussions of experimental findings by various workers and also the sources of error in the studies, they state: "Experiments described show that alcohol is oxidized in the body, and that its potential energy thus becomes kinetic and is utilized in various ways. In these respects alcohol is more or less similar to the few ingredients of ordinary food, i.e. the carbohydrates and fat. The nutritive action of alcohol may, for our present purpose, be called its direct action. It is equally well established, indeed, the fact has been much longer known, that alcohol has a very different action, exercised partly or wholly through the nervous system, of which the most familiar form found is drunkenness. It is believed that in this pharmacodynamic action alcohol exercises a very important influence upon metabolism. This may be called its indirect action, as contracted with its direct action just referred to. From the standpoint of the pharmacologist, this pharmacodynamic action would perhaps be called its direct action, but it is termed indirect because we're discussing the subject from the standpoint of nutritive value. We have thus a very clear distinction between alcohol as food and alcohol as drug. The failure to observe this distinction has led to errors in the planning of experiments and serious confusion in the discussion of results."

In order to justify further studies to find out about the nutritional properties of alcohol, Atwater, in his major report, cites cases in which alcohol was used as the only "food" over a period of time. One of these was a girl in the Massachusetts General Hospital with pneumonia, who received more than a gallon of brandy and whiskey over a period of seven days and no other form of food or drugs.

Atwater's studies were carried out over the years 1898 to 1900 in the chemical laboratory of Wesleyan University. Normal, young male subjects, some of them laboratory workers, participated in metabolic studies in which they were fed diets of known macronutrient content with/without alcohol. The subjects performed standard work upon a stationary bicycle inside the large respiration calorimeter and the heat given off by each subject was measured.

The major conclusions derived from these studies are that in human subjects alcohol is oxidized in the body and serves as a fuel. Further, any nutrients, according to these investigators, serving as fuel protect or, as we should say, spare one another. Thus, they suggest that alcohol spares protein and fat and possibly also carbohydrates. Finally, they consider from the results of their investigations, that alcohol resembles ordinary foods with respect to its oxidation. It differs from foods in that it is not held in the body for any considerable time for future use (Billings, 1903).

Prior to the completion of Atwater's studies, an editorial appeared in the Journal of The American Medical Association entitled "Alcohol as A Food" (1900). Opening statements of this editorial show the support and approbation with which Atwater's findings were received in 1900: "The Temperance workers of the W.C.T.U. are somewhat agitated over the alledged statement of Professor Atwater, that alcohol is a food and that therefore teachings of the physiologic textbooks to the contrary are incorrect. The antitemperance people are correspondingly elated by his findings and make the most of them. It seems to us that there is as little basis for alarm on the one hand as for elation on the other, especially when Professor Atwater has expressly said that he believed alcohol an excellent thing for healthy persons to let alone. The whole agitation depends upon the signification of the word 'food.' If it means anything that is oxidized and used up to any extent in the human body, it will include a very great many unwholesome, unpleasant substances besides alcohol. A man can support life on carrion..."

It is interesting that in the same volume of the Journal of The American Medical Association there is an article by a medical temperance supporter, T.D. Crothers (1900). He comments, "From a pathological point of view, alcohol is shown to be one of the most insidious and destructive of tissue poisons and its use followed by certain cell and tissue degenerations that are uniform in their progress and growth. The theory of atonic and stimulant value or a producer or food conserver cannot be sustained by any facts that are unquestioned."

Arguments about the nutritional value of alcohol persisted for many years, and during Prohibition, whereas the "drys" justified campaigns to make alcohol therapeutically unfashionable, the "wets" called attention to the value of alcohol for nourishment as well as a stimulant to appetite (Jones, 1963).

Today such arguments about the nutritional therapeutic properties of alcohol can still raise voices. However, current medical opinion is perhaps best stated by Becker *et al.* who wrote in 1974: "Alcohol has been used clinically as an appetite stimulant, as a sedative-hypnotic drug and as a calorie source for intravenous alimentation. Such medicinal uses of alcohol have never been subjected to controlled evaluation. Many health tonics contain substantial quantities of alcohol and may as a consequence be abused."

SELECTED REFERENCES

Allen, W. 1736. *Ways and Means to Raise the Value of Land.* London.

Anon. 1900. Editorial. J. Amer. Med. Assoc. 34: 302-303.

Anstie, F.E. 1864. *Stimulants and Narcotics.* London. p. 489.

Anstie, F.E. 1974. Final experiments on the elimination of alcohol from the body. Practitioner 73: 15-28.

Anstie, F.E. 1877. *On the Uses of Wine in Health and Disease.* Macmillan and Co., Ltd., London.

Antal, F. 1952. *The Moral Purpose of Hogarth's Art.* J. Warburg and Courtauld Institutes 15: 161-197.

Arderne, J. 1922. *"De Arte Phisicale et de Cirurgia" of Master John Arderne, Surgeon of Newark, 1412.* Trans. D'Arcy Power, Early English Text Society, London. Vol. 2, p. 17.

Atwater, W.O. and Benedict, F.B. 1900. Experiments on the metabolism of matter and energy in the human body. Bulls. #69, 109, USDA, Washington D.C.

Atwater, W.O., Woods, C.D. and Benedict, F.G. 1903. Report of preliminary investigations on the metabolism of nitrogen and carbons in the human organism with a respiration calorimeter of special construction. Bull. #44, Ofc. of Experiment Stations of U.S.D.A., Washington, D.C.

Aylward, F. 1972. Alcohol consumption in its different forms. Proc. Nutr. Soc. 31: 77-82.

Becker, C.E., Roe, R.L. and Scott, R.A. 1974. *Alcohol as a Drug: A Curriculum on Pharmacology, Neurology and Toxicology.* Baltimore: The Williams and Wilkins Co.

Benezet. 1774. *The Potent Enemies of America Laid Open - Being Some Account of the Bainful Effects Attending Use of Distilled Spiritous Liquors and the Slavery of Negroes. The Mighty Destroyer Displayed in Some Account of the Dreadful Havoc Made by the Mistaken Use as Well as Abuse of Distilled Spiritous Liquors. By a Lover of Mankind.* Collected by Anthony Benezet. Philadelphia: J. Crukshank.

Bentley Todd, R. 1860. *Clinical Lectures on Certain Acute Diseases. Lecture 14 on the Therapeutic Action of Alcohol.* London.

Billings, J.S., ed. 1903. The nutritive value of alcohol. IN *Psychological Aspects of the Liquor Problem.* Vol. 2. Boston and New York: Horton, Mifflin and Co. (The Univ. Press, Cambridge). pp. 174-343.

Blane, G. 1785. *Observations on the Diseases of Seamen.* London: J. Cooper. pp. 282, 293.

Bourne, P.G. 1973. Alcoholism in the urban Negro population. IN *Alcoholism. Progress in Research and Treatment.* Eds. Bourne, P.G. and Fox, R. New York and London: Academic Press. pp. 211-226.

Bruhl-Cramer. 1819. Ueber Trunksucht. Berlin.

Bynum, W.F. 1968. Chronic alcoholism in the first half of the 19th century. Bull. Hist. Med. 42: 160-185.

Cockayne, T.O. 1864-6. Leechdoms, Wortcunning and Starcraft in Early England I: 75; III: 117. Rolls Series, London.

Catalog of Prints and Drawings of the British Museum 1934. Vol 3, Part 1, #2277. London: Chissick Press.

Chalke, H.D. 1976. Alcohol and history. Brit. J. Alcohol and Alcoholism 11: 128-149.

Coffey, T.G. 1966. Beer Street; Gin Lane. Some views of 18th century drinking. Quart. J. Stud. Alc. 27: 669-692.

Crothers, T.D. 1900. Continental views of alcohol in therapeutics. J. Amer. Med. Assoc. 34: 26-28.

Darby, W.J., Ghalioungui, P. and Grivetti, L. 1977. *Food: The Gift of Osiris.* Vol 2. London, New York, San Francisco: Academic Press. pp. 529-595.

Davenant, C. 1695. *An Essay Upon Ways and Means of Supplying the War.* London. p. 138.

Dorothy George, M. 1925. 1st Ed. *London Life in the 18th Century.* Kegan Paul, Trench, Trubner and Co., Ltd. 2nd Ed. 1966, London: Peregrine Books. pp. 42-43.

Dorothy George, M. 1931. *England in Transition. Life and Work in the 18th Century.* London: G. Routledge and Sons, Ltd. p. 93.

Dupré, A. 1871-2. On the elimination of alcohol. Proc. Roy. Soc. London 20, p. 268.

Dupré, A. 1872. The physiological action of alcohol - an answer to Dr. Subbotin. Practitioner 148: p. 8.

Fielding, H. 1751. *An Enquiry into the Causes of the Late Increase of Robbers, etc. With Some Proposals for Remedying the Evil. Dedicated to the Right Honourable Philip, Lord Hardwick, Lord High Chancellor of Great Britain.* Section II, Drunkenness. p. 20.

French, R.V. 1891. *Nineteen Centuries of Drink in England.* 2nd ed. Nat. Temperance Publ. Depot.

Fuchs, C.H. 1848. *Lehrbuch der Speciellen Pathologie und Terapie.* Vol. 2. Gottingen. pp. 937-951.

Gower, J. 1881. Confessio Amantis. Book 6, pp. 26-75, quoted in French, R.V. *History of Toasting or Drinking of Healths in England.* National Temperance Publ. Depot, London.

Hirsch, J. 1949. Enlightened 18th century views of the alcohol problem. J. Hist. Med. 4: 230-236.

Horsley, V. and Sturge, M. 1907. *Alcohol and the Human Body.* Macmillan and Co. Ltd., London, 1908. (1st ed. 1907).

Huss, M. 1852. *Chronische Alkoholkrankheit Oder Alcoholismus Chronicus.* Van den Busch, Stockholm and Leipzig.

Hutchison, R. 1905. *Food and the Principles of Dietetics.* New York: W. Wood Co. pp. 335, 464-466.

Jellinek, E.M. 1942. *Alcohol Addiction and Chronic Alcoholism.* Yale Univ. Press, New Haven. Vol. 1.

Jolliffe, N. 1940. The influence of alcohol on the adequacy of the B vitamins in the American diet. Quart. J. Stud. Alc. 1: 74-84.

Jones, B.C. 1963. A Prohibition problem. Liquor as medicine, 1920-1933. J. Hist. Med. 18: 353-369.

Korsakoff, S.S. 1889. Psychosis polyneuritica s cerebropathia psychica toxaemica. Med. Obozr. Mosk. 32: 3-18.

Lallemand, L., Perrin, M. and Duroy, J.-L.P. 1860. *Du Role de L'alcool et des Anestesiques Dans L'organisme, Recherches Experimentales.* Paris. L

Lettsom, J.C. 1786. *Some Remarks on the Effects of Lignum Quassiae Amarae.* Lecture Med. Soc. London.

Lettsom, J.C. 1792. History of some of the effects of hard drinking. Memoirs Med. Soc. London 1: 128-165.

Lord Kinross 1959. Prohibition in Britain. History Today 9: 493-499.

Lucia, S.P. 1963. The Antiquity of Alcohol in Diet and Medicine. IN *Alcohol and Civilization,* ed. Lucia S.P. New York, San Francisco, Toronto, London: McGraw-Hill Book Co., Inc. pp. 171-172.

Martindale, M. 1972. *The Extra Pharmacopaeia.* 26th ed. London: Pharmaceutical Press. p. 50.

Minot, G.R., Strauss, M.B. and Cobb, S. 1933. "Alcoholic" polyneuritis; dietary deficiency as a factor in its production. New Eng. J. Med. 208: 1244-1249.

Packowski, George, W. 1974. Distilled Beverage Spirits. *In Encyclopedia of Food Technology.* A.H. Johnson and M.S. Peterson (Editors). AVI Publishing Co., Westport, Conn.

Rix, K.J.B. 1975. James Boswell (1740-1795). J. Alcoholism 10: 73-77.

Rix, K.J.B. 1976. John Coakley Lettsom and some effects of hard drinking. J. Alcoholism 11: 97-103.

Rolleston, J.D. 1927. Alcoholism in classical antiquity. Brit. J. Inebriety 24: 101-120.

Rolleston, J.D. 1928. Alcohol in acute infectious diseases. Brit. J. Inebriety 25: 201-203.

Rolleston, J.D. 1929. Alcohol in therapeutics. Brit. J. Inebriety 27: 1-13.

Rolleston, J.D. 1933a. Alcoholism in medieval England. Brit. J. Inebriety 31: 33-49.

Rolleston, J.D. 1933b. *Alcohol in Medical Practice, 1832-1932.* Nat. Temperance Soc. Reprint.

Rolleston, J.D. 1941. The folklore of alcoholism. Brit. J. Inebriety, Reprint.

Rolleston, J.D. 1944. Peyps and alcoholism. Brit. J. Inebriety, Reprint Jan.-April.

Rush, B. 1809. *Medical Inquiries and Observations.* Philadelphia: M. Carey and Son. 5th ed., Vol. 1, 1818.

Rush, B. 1943. Inquiry into the Effects of Ardent Spirits upon the Human Body and Mind. Reprinted Quart. J. Studies Alcohol 4: 321-28.

Sedgwick, J. 1725. *A New Treatise on Liquors Wherein the Use and Abuse of Wine, Malt Drinks, Water, Etc. Are Particularly Considered in Many Diseases, Constitutions and Ages with the Proper Manner of Using Them Hot or Cold Either as Physick, Diet or Both.* Rivington, London.

Singer, N., Holmyard, E.J. Hall, A.R. and Williams, T.I., Eds. 1956. *A History of Technology.* Oxford: Clarendon Press. Vol. 2.

Smith, E. 1887. *A Practical Treatise on Disease in Children.* 3rd ed., J. & A. Churchill, pp. 18, 641, 645. (First ed. 1884).

Thudichum, J.L.W. 1868. *A Consideration of the Amount of Alcohol Eliminated After the Ingestion of Alcoholic Drinks. Appendix #7.* 10th Report of the Medical Officer of the Privy Council, London, p. 295.

Trotter, T. 1804. *An Essay, Medical, Philosophical, and Chemical on Drunkenness and its Effects on the Human Body.* London: Longman, Hurst, Rees and Orme. 2nd ed., pp. 97-136.

Tucker, B.R. 1911. Pellagra, with the analytical study of 55 non-institutional or sporadic cases. J. Amer. Med. Assoc. 56: 246-255.

Webb, S. and Webb, B. 1903. *The History of Liquor Licensing in England, Principally from 1700 to 1830.* London, New York and Bombay: Longmans, Green & Co.

Wheatley, H.B. 1909. *Hogarth's London. Pictures of the Manners of the 18th Century.* New York: E.P. Dutton and Sons. p. 156.

Winskill, P.T. 1881. *The Comprehensive History of the Rise and Progress of Temperance Reformation—from the Earliest Period to September 1881.* Crewe, England: Mackie, Brewtnall and Co.

Wilson, T. 1736. *Distilled Spiritous Liquors - the Bane of the Nation: Being Some Considerations Humbly Offer'd to the Legislature.* 2nd Ed. London.

Zirker, M.R. 1966. *Fielding's Social Pamphlets.* Berkeley, Los Angeles: Univ. California Press. pp. 88-91.

2

Alcohol and Appetite

In any discussion of the effects of alcohol on food intake, distinction must be made between effects of alcohol ingestion on the physiological and behavioral indicators that food is needed. It is therefore appropriate to seek some definitions. Le Gros Clark (1968) distinguishes between appetite and "being hungry" and between repletion and satiety: "Appetite," he states, "is not quite the same as being unreplete. We observe it as a group of sensations responsive to savor and expected taste, and identify it with labial and palatal stimuli, a slight emission of saliva...Appetite often works independently of repletion...It is not necessarily a guide to sufficiency in food intake." Le Gros Clark indicates that repletion relates to the gastric and visceral warnings that we have eaten enough and that satiety according to this author is a term to be used for eating to the level of discomfort. It is suggested then that hunger should be the reverse of repletion, or that it is a term to cover the physiological and not the behavioral indicators of immediate requirement for food. In any population, there are those people whose food intake is mainly conditioned by hunger, and others in whom food intake is conditioned more by appetite: that is, they will only eat if the food is appealing to them. Le Gros Clark suggests that people responding to hunger are mainly those who are conditioned to eat a monotonous diet and people engaged in heavy manual work. Such people stop eating at a stage of repletion.

For most people in our industrialized society, eating as well as drinking is highly influenced by appetite or the sensory appeal of food. There is very strong evidence that in certain segments of the population another factor aside from hunger and appetite may influence food as well as alcohol intake, and that is boredom. Eating or drinking is a fine way of passing time, particularly for those whose lives are dull, depressing or attended by social failure.

We should separately consider the effects of alcohol on hunger, appetite and the boredom-eating factor.

ALCOHOL AND HUNGER

The effect of alcohol on the sensation of hunger was investigated and reported in 1938 by Scott *et al.* They determined the effect of ingestion of 200 ml of 20% alcohol, taken in two 100 ml doses 5 minutes apart on hunger contractions, and hunger sense, in six healthy males. Stomach motility was inhibited for an average of 50 minutes following this dose of alcohol but after this time the sensation of hunger was increased in all subjects, an increased desire for food developing within five minutes after ingesting the alcohol.

Several authors have studied gastric motility and gastric emptying time after alcohol ingestion in human subjects. It has been concluded that dilute alcohol solutions increase while concentrated solutions decrease gastric motility. Gastric emptying time is delayed by alcohol ingestion, but no correlation has been obtained between the delay in gastric emptying and the concentration of the alcohol. Beazell and Ivy (1940) in reviewing these and other studies of the effects of alcohol on the digestive tract, conclude that the increase in appetite which has been ascribed to the intake of alcoholic drinks, is due to the stimulation of taste and other oral sensations as well as to a central effect with the promotion of a general sense of well being, and hence, a desire for food. They note that these stimulatory effects of alcohol on appetite occur with small doses whereas with larger intakes of alcohol, hunger may be depressed.

EATING HABITS AMONG DRINKERS

Decreased desire for food in heavy drinkers may be due to associated habits including coffee drinking and smoking. Correlations between cigarette smoking, consumption of coffee and alcohol have been reported by several authors (Friedman *et al.*, 1974; Heath, 1958; Higgins, 1967; and Matarazzo and Saslow, 1960). A need for cigarettes and coffee is often claimed by people with anxiety neuroses who also indulge in binge drinking. While hunger may be reduced by constant smoking, disinclination for food in those who cannot resist coffee, cigarettes, or alcohol may be another manifestation of their neurosis.

Studies of alcohol consumers who are not alcoholics do not suggest that their drinking practices reduce food intake. Bebb *et al.* (1971) studied men and women with multiple sclerosis as well as normal men in executive, management or professional positions with respect to their food and alcohol consumption. There was a progressive increase in the average daily energy intake as the percent of total energy intake from alcohol increased. Among the male alcohol consumers in the study, the mean caloric intake for non-drinking days was similar to that of men who reported no alcohol intake during the study. In the women, caloric intakes for the drinkers on non-drinking days was higher than that of the women who consumed no alcohol. For each group of subjects, the total caloric intake on drinking days was higher than on days when no alcohol was taken. Weight gain was not related to alcohol consumption in this sample population. Lack of significant weight gain when additional calories were consumed from alcohol may have one of two explanations: in the first place, 73 of the 155 subjects in the study had multiple sclerosis with various degrees of disability, which could have been associated with a catabolic state. Another possibility is that the alcohol consumers did, in fact, experience some reduction in appetite and did consume less food because of greater plate waste. This matter is not discussed by the authors, nor is there any description of the patient's subjective ratings of appetite or hunger on drinking versus non-drinking days.

In a more recent study, reported from Finland by Hasunen *et al.* (1976), dietary intakes of men with high alcohol consumption patterns were compared with intakes of a control group in a normal population. The control group consisted of men either who did not drink, or who had a low alcohol consumption. Dietary information was obtained by diet history using a standardized questionnaire. Mean intakes of absolute alcohol in the high alcohol consumption group were more than 30 gm/day. The food consumption in weight of the high alcohol group was greater than that of the low alcohol control group. These differences were reduced when consumption figures were expressed as an energy unit. Nutrient consumption patterns between the high and low alcohol group were different. The high alcohol group obtained more fats and less carbohydrates in relation to their total intake of energy than the low alcohol groups, and intakes of calcium, vitamin A and riboflavin were lower in the high alcohol group than the control group.

Traditionally, alcoholics have been considered to fall into two groups: those who eat and drink and grow fat, and those who drink and don't eat and get thin. Such a superficial approach to the problem of food intake in the alcoholic is factual but fails to explain why or when alcoholics eat normally or to excess, and when their appetite and their food intake is diminished. Until recent years, loss of appetite in the alcoholic was seen to have one major cause—namely satiety due to

TABLE 2.1. RELATIONSHIPS BETWEEN DRINKING AND EATING.

Percent of Irish-Americans and Italian-Americans by Country of Birth Who Drink in Selected Contexts:[a]

	Irish-Americans USA	Italian-Americans USA	Italy
At a wedding	92	93	93
On family occasions	84	90	93
At a party	87	91	87
When visiting a friend's home	82	85	87
At a bar with a friend	71	72	67
At home alone	40	38	55
At a bar alone	33	20	32
At meals	44	59	87

Percent of Teenage Drinkers in Rome and New York by Age and Context:[a]

	Rome 13-15 yrs.	16-20 yrs.	New York 13-15 yrs.	16-20 yrs.
At home	95	93	74	22
Parties at home	4	0	24	5
Special family events	33	56	24	6
Parties away from home	53	67	42	51
With friends	21	30	33	38
With dates	0	0	3	17
Alone*	50	20	0	11.5
Breakfast	26	10	2	0
Lunch	73	79	0	0
Dinner	64	71	42	49
Afternoon	63	56	26	11
Evening	31	53	43	97

*Drinking alone entailed circumstances of meals separated from other members of the family and involved the use of wine for the Italian sample.

/Alcohol & Health. USDHEW Public Health Service, Second Special Report to the U.S. Congress. June, 1974, Washington, D.C. (M. Keller, editor)

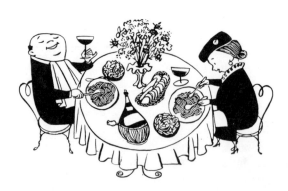

From "Facts about Alcohol," by R.G. McCarthy. Science Research Associates, Inc., 47 W. Grand Ave., Chicago, IL, 1951.

intake of "food" in the form of alcoholic beverages. In his discussion of alcohol addicts, Olsen (1950) states:

... There is poor intake of food, vomiting and diarrhea. Most of the calories consumed are obtained from the non-nutritional alcoholic beverages ... in the alcoholic a high intake of such calories contributes to a poor appetite.

While this author also considered that gastrointestinal abnormalities including gastritis and enteritis might cause anorexia, he was clearly of the opinion that a reduced appetite for food was mainly due to the concurrent intake of energy from alcohol sources.

NUTRITIONAL CAUSES OF ANOREXIA

In experimental animals and, to a lesser extent, in human subjects, nutrient imbalances in the diet as well as nutritional deficiencies may be associated with loss of appetite. Marginal diets, low in B vitamins and protein, consumed by indigent chronic alcoholics, may cause a reduction in food intake. Deficiencies of several B vitamins induce anorexia, but of these, the most constant cause is a thiamin deficiency. Acute thiamin deficiency causes anorexia. In a 1945 research report by Keys on the effect of acute deprivation of B vitamins, the development of anorexia with B vitamin restriction and more particularly, thiamin restriction, is recorded. The experimental design as well as the description of the development of anorexia in study subjects can be used as an analogy with the course of events which may pertain in an alcoholic. Eight normal young men subsisted for 32 days on a diet which was adequate except in B vitamins which were very limited (thiamin 0.008 mg/day; riboflavin 0.013 mg/day; niacin 0.1 mg/1000 cal.). Energy intake and expenditure were set at 4,000 Kcal daily. Half of these men had been on a somewhat B vitamin-restricted diet for six months prior to the study. The other men had received the same diet with the addition of a B vitamin supplement to the level of the then National Research Council Recommended Allowances. In the second portion of the study, half of the men were given a B vitamin supplement. There were therefore four groups of men according to diet: the restricted-deficient, the control-deficient, the restricted-control and the control-control; this separation being made on the basis of the first and second diets. Anorexia, followed by nausea and vomiting, began in the restricted-deficient men after about eight days, and developed very rapidly so that they were unable to eat in about 18-20 days. The control-deficient men showed anorexia but with a lag period of 5-6 days. After 22 days the men in both of these groups were given daily supplements with thiamin and their appetites returned and the other symptoms of nausea and vomiting ceased. It is of interest that the men on the restricted-deficient and control-deficient diets showed psychological changes including apathy, depression and hypochondriasis.

Several questions must be answered here with respect to the association between alcoholism, thiamin deficiency and anorexia. Are alcoholics, subsisting on a diet low in B vitamins, more vulnerable to develop thiamin deficiency when supply of the vitamin is further reduced below the level of requirements? Further, is lack of desire for food conditioned by apathy and the other emotional responses to thiamin deficiency? This situation may be the outcome of prolonged drinking sprees in chronic alcoholics, particularly those with psychotic depression.

Thiamin deficiency syndromes in alcoholics have been variously attributed to inadequate intake of the vitamin, impaired absorption or defective utilization. While according to Figueroa et al. (1953) the incidence of alcoholic neuropathies and encephalopathies, directly attributable either to thiamin deficiency per se or to mixed B vitamin deficiencies has been markedly reduced in the U.S. since the general practice of fortifying bread and cereals with B vitamins was adopted in 1943, the risk of thiamin deficiency remains due to thiamin malabsorption and particularly because alcoholics may become thiamin-dependent in that their requirements for the vitamin are higher than in normal individuals. Thiamin deficiency in alcoholics has also been attributed to defects in the metabolism of the vitamin (Sauberlich, 1967).

The relationship of thiamin deficiency to anorexia in alcoholics is complex. Anorexia, or refusal to eat, associated with thiamin deficiency, may in itself have several etiologies. Thiamin deficiency does not only cause anorexia because of the accompanying nausea, or because of apathy and depression. If an alcoholic eats a thiamin-deficient diet, food intake could be reduced because such a diet is monotonous (Berryman et al., 1947). Neurological complications of thiamin deficiency in the alcoholic including Wernicke's encephalopathy, explains refusal to eat because affected patients are drowsy and confused (Hunter, 1976 and Victor, 1960).

ANOREXIC EFFECTS OF OTHER B VITAMIN DEFICIENCIES

Vitamin B6 deficiency has been found in alcoholics with decompensated cirrhosis. Apparently this is not due to a deficient intake of the vitamin, but rather to an increased rate of pyridoxal phosphate degradation (Labadarios et al.,1957). Anorexia, nausea, vomiting and drowsiness occur in experimental vitamin B6 deficiency, and it is possible that when these symptoms occur in the alcoholic with cirrhosis, they may also be due to vitamin B6 deficiency (Vilter, 1953).

Pellagra, now an uncommon disease in alcoholics, causes loss of appetite or refusal to eat because niacin deficiency induces severe glossitis and also because of the accompanying confusional psychosis (Wood, 1912).

LOSS OF TASTE IN ZINC DEFICIENCY

Zinc deficiency, associated with hyperzincuria and abnormal zinc utilization, has commonly been found in alcoholics with cirrhosis. These patients with zinc deficiency are markedly anorectic (Sullivan and Lankford, 1965; and Vallee et al., 1957). Zinc deficiency is associated not only with anorexia, but also decreased taste acuity in human subjects. The reduced sense of smell may also occur with zinc deficiency, and may precede loss of taste in the development of the depletion state. While it is not justifiable to assume that these abnormalities of taste and smell are always due to zinc deficiency, taste perversions may occur in hepatitis, including alcoholic hepatitis, and abnormalities of taste and smell occur in cirrhosis (Cohen et al., 1973; and Sullivan and Birch, 1976). It is true that if food loses its savor to the alcoholic in terms both of its aroma and taste, intake may be severely curtailed. In addition, if zinc supplements are given orally to alcoholics exhibiting loss of taste and smell as well as biochemical evidence of zinc deficiency, the sensory abnormality is reversed and appetite will improve (personal communication). However, if the zinc deficient or cirrhotic patient, on medical advice, consumes a low protein diet, this may reduce a desire for food, particularly if the diet is bland and unsalted, because taste cannot be appreciated.

AVERSIVE RESPONSES TO FOOD INTAKE

If food intake is repeatedly followed by unpleasant symptoms, then the tendency is to reduce the amount eaten to a point where these symptoms may be avoided or minimized. In the alcoholic, aversive symptoms after eating are mainly related to the following gastro-intestinal disorders.

1. Gastritis

Acute gastritis follows episodic drinking and is due to gastric mucosal injury induced by the alcohol (Chey, 1972). Symptoms may begin while drinking is going on, or may be delayed until the drinking bout is over. Appetite is completely lost and thirst is excessive. The patient repeatedly belches, and vomiting is likely to occur preceded by nausea. Food eaten immediately prior to the drinking episode, or during the period of drinking, is rejected and vomitus contains mucus and later bile. The tongue is furred and there is an unpleasant, bitter taste in the mouth. Upper abdominal pain, a sensation of fullness or epigastric discomfort, as well as epigastric tenderness, supervene rapidly (Price, 1944).

During the period of drunkenness all food may be refused, but after the drinker sleeps off his/her excesses, small amounts of certain foods may be accepted on the supposition that they will not induce vomiting or exacerbate abdominal discomfort. Foods are often selected by sensory acceptability and may include apples, chicken, sherbet, and jels. Thirst may be marked due to dehydration. A craving for salt is often described in episodic drinkers following binges. Recovery generally takes place in 24 hours or less, but symptoms may persist for several days. Effects of binge drinking on nutrient intake can be substantial if the episodes are frequent, or if drinking goes on for periods up to a week or more.

Chronic gastritis is the outcome of long-term alcohol abuse. As with acute gastritis, it is due to the direct toxic effect of the alcohol on the stomach and is not mediated by malnutrition, liver damage or anemia. Alcohol abuse is frequently associated with heavy smoking and each of these toxic substances can cause chronic gastritis and if both alcoholic excess and smoking occur together, then there may be an additive or synergistic effect. Although malnutrition may occur in alcoholics with chronic gastritis, the gastric pathology is apparently not associated with dyspeptic symptoms and has a variable and perhaps insignificant effect on food intake (Roberts, 1972). If alcoholics with chronic gastitis do have a decreased food intake, it is more likely to be due to associated cigarette smoking, which is well known as a cause of diminished food intake (Batterman, 1955; and Pawan, 1974).

Whereas it is not confirmed that acute or chronic gastritis are precursors to the development of gastric ulcer, the association of alcoholic gastritis with gastric ulcer may intensify ulcer symptoms and thereby reduce food intake. Association of pain with meal eating in the ulcer patient may lead the patient to reduced intake, though no actual anorexia is present. It has been suggested (Friedman *et al.,* 1974) that a failure to correlate ulcer symptoms with alcohol ingestion and reduced food intake may be due to a general tendency for patients with peptic ulcer to cut down on alcohol consumption.

2. Postgastrectomy Syndromes

Among peptic ulcer patients who have undergone partial gastrectomy, alcoholics are over-represented. The association between continued alcohol excess and reduced appetite associated with postgastrectomy syndromes have a devastating effect on nutritional status (Nilsson and Westlin, 1972). Causes of inadequate food intake after gastrectomy include diminished appetite, a feeling of fullness and early satiety, as well as fear of post-cibal symptoms such as regurgitation and the dumping syndrome. Other factors cited as etiologically related to reduced appetite after gastrectomy include superficial gastritis and chronic iron deficiency. Diarrhea may also occur following ingestion of food, thus discouraging the patient from eating (Alexander, 1965).

3. Disaccharide Intolerance

Recent studies by Perlow *et al.* (1977) have indicated that chronic alcohol ingestion decreases the activity of intestinal disaccharidases, particularly lactase activity. Lactase activity was less than 1 U/g in 100% of black and 20% of white alcoholics as compared to 50% of the black and none of the white control subjects. Alcohol abstinence led to a return or partial return in activity of the disaccharidase activity. Lactose malabsorption, particularly in black alcoholics, following ingestion of milk, was associated with colicky pain, diarrhea and sometimes a dumping-like syndrome. It is conceived that the alcoholic, knowing that milk or foods containing milk will evoke unpleasant symptoms, may well refrain from eating or drinking such foods.

4. Pancreatitis

Both acute and chronic pancreatitis are variously associated with alcohol excess. In considering associations between acute pancreatitis and reduced food intake, it is important to understand that mild and subclinical but repeated attacks of acute pancreatitis may follow binge drinking episodes. Dreiling *et al.* (1952) in reviewing the association between alcoholism and pancreatitis, point out that attacks may follow not only high intake of alcohol, but also a heavy meal. A patient with mild to moderate acute pancreatitis may come to associate attacks of abdominal colic, often radiating with the back, with consumption of large meals and may therefore reduce intake in order to try to avoid recurrence of the pain. Alternately, the pain may be severe enough to stop the patient from eating during the attacks. Chronic pancreatitis is also associated with abdominal pain and with periodic diarrhea, characterized by the production of large, foul stools. The patient may reduce food intake or fat intake because he/she comes to associate eating fatty foods either with exacerbation of abdominal pain or with worsening of the diarrhea. Painful episodes may also cause nausea and vomiting as well as anorexia (Kowlessar, 1963).

5. Alcoholic Hepatitis

The clinical symptoms of alcoholic hepatitis are quite variable. Complaints of anorexia are common but not uniform, and the degree to which anorexia interferes with food intake varies with the patient characteristics as well as the severity of the disease (Helman *et al.* 1969; and Lischner *et al.*, 1971). As in viral hepatitis, loss of appetite may precede the development of jaundice or may occur in subicteric cases. Jaundice is often accompanied by nausea and vomiting may be troublesome. When alcoholic hepatitis is attended by impending hepatocellular failure, an unwillingness to accept food may be due to mental confusion.

6. Laennec's Cirrhosis

Reduced caloric intakes are common in patients with alcoholic cirrhosis. Patek *et al.* (1975) studied the dietary intakes of alcoholics with and without cirrhosis. Records of food intake were obtained for a period of at least two years before the presenting illness, and were corroborated by the patients' families. Although there were no statistically significant differences between alcoholics without cirrhosis, those with a precirrhotic condition, or those with frank cirrhosis with respect to the amount of alcohol drunk, cirrhotics had lower energy intakes than non-cirrhotics. Medical factors contributing to poor food intakes in alcoholics with cirrhosis include ascites or dyspnea, evoked by meal eating, in a patient with gross ascitic distension of the abdomen. Food intake may be reduced in order to avoid respiratory embarrassment. In patients with cirrhosis, anorexia may also, as previously suggested, be due to zinc deficiency with loss of taste.

7. Early Satiety

Another factor contributing to poor food intake is early satiety. Palasciano *et al.* (1974) have demonstrated that chronic ethanol feeding augments the cholecystokinin (CCK) releasing capacity of the duodenal mucosa. CCK release acts as a satiety signal. Effects of alcohol may therefore augment the short term satiety via the CCK mechanism (Smith *et al.,* 1974).

8. Alcoholic Ketoacidosis

Levy *et al.* (1973) identified a condition of ketoacidosis in chronic alcoholics who had recently been on drinking sprees. Symptoms preceeding or associated with the development of severe ketoacidosis were protracted vomiting and abstention from food. Anorexia was the rule. Acidosis was associated with accumulation of β-hydroxybutyrate, acetoacetate and lactate in the blood plasma. Circulating levels of free fatty acids were high. Ketone body synthesis was believed to be due to enhanced release of free fatty acids from adipose tissue stores. The authors thought that lipolysis could be secondary to increased concentrations of plasma cortisol and growth hormone, or perhaps other lipolytic hormones. Other authors (Petersen, 1973) recorded the same syndrome which is apparently a cause as well as an effect of anorexia in the alcoholic.

SOCIAL AND BEHAVIORAL FACTORS INFLUENCING FOOD INTAKE IN ALCOHOLICS

Inadequate living arrangements, marital separations, economic privation and a vagrant life count for inadequate food intake among the skid-row group of alcoholics (Ashley *et al.*, 1976). When alcohol is taken with food, a central nervous system effect is less than when the same quantity of alcohol is taken on an empty stomach. Mellanby (1920) showed that after eating at the same time as drinking, there were reduced concentrations of ethanol in the blood.

Because food delays gastric emptying and decreases the rate of alcohol absorption, lower blood alcohol levels may result. According to Sedman *et al.* (1976), not only is the rate of alcohol absorption slowed by food intake, but also the relative efficiency of alcohol metabolism is increased.

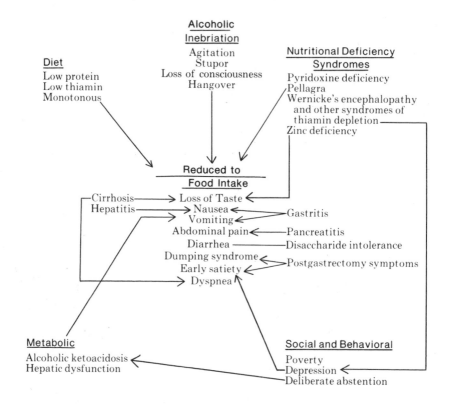

FIG 2.1
SUMMARY OF FACTORS CONTRIBUTING TO REDUCED FOOD INTAKE

It has been suggested that alcoholics who wish to get drunk quickly may purposefully refrain from eating. An alcoholic subject studied by Mello (1972) commented that he intended at one point to stop eating in order to increase the effects of his alcohol. Reduction in food intake in this case led to a three-fold increase in blood alcohol levels. In discussing this case, the author postulates that alcoholics do learn that eating less food effectively enhances intoxicating properties of a given amount of alcohol (Mello and Mendelson, 1970).

SELECTED REFERENCES

Alexander Williams, J. 1965. The long term metabolic effects of partial gastrectomy. IN *Recent Advances in Gastroenterology*. Eds. Badenoch, J. and Brooke, B.N. J&A Churchill Ltd.: London. pp 86-106.

Ashley, M.J., Olin, J.S., Harding Le Riche, W., Kornaczewski, A., Schmidt, W. and Rankin, J.G. 1976. Skid row alcoholism: A distinct socio-medical entity. Arch. Intern. Med. 136: 272-278.

Batterman, R.L. 1955. IN *The Biological Effects of Tobacco*. Ed. Wynder, E.L. Boston, Mass: Little & Brown. p. 140.

Beazell, J.M. and Ivy, A.C. 1940. The influence of alcohol on the digestive tract. Quart. J. Stud. Alc. 1: 45-73.

Bebb, H.T., Houser, H.B., Witschi, J.C., Littell, A.S. and Fuller, R.K. 1971. Calorie and nutrient contribution of alcoholic beverages to the usual diets of 155 adults. Am.J. Clin. Nutr. 24: 1042-1052.

Berryman, G.H. *et al.* 1947. Effects in young men consuming restricted quantities of B-complex vitamins and proteins and changes associated with supplementation. Amer. J. Physiol. 148: 618-646.

Chey, W.Y. 1972. Alcohol and gastric mucosa. Digestion 7: 239-251.

Cohen, I.K., Schechter, P.J. and Henkin, R.I. 1973. Hypogeusia, anorexia, and altered zinc metabolism following thermal burn. J. Am. Med. S. 223: 914-916.

Dreiling, D.A., Richman, A., and Fradkin, N.F. 1952. The role of alcohol in the etiology of pancreatitis: A study of the effect of intravenous ethyl alcohol on the external secretion of the pancreas. Gastroenterology 20: 636-646.

Figueroa, W.G., Sargent, F., Imperiale, L., Morey, G.R., Paynter, C.R., Vorhaurs, L.I. and Kark, R. M. 1953. Lack of avitaminosis among alcoholics: Its relation to fortification of cereal products and the general nutritional status of the population. J. Clin. Nutr. 1: 179-199.

Friedman, G.D., Sieglaub, A.B. and Seltzer, C.C. 1974. Cigarettes, alcohol, coffee and peptic ulcer. New Eng. J. Med. 290: 469-473.

Hasunen, K., Pekkarinen, M. and Nuutinen, O. 1976. Alcohol consumption and dietary intake of Finnish men. Nutr. Metab. 20: 176 (Abst.).

Heath, C.W. 1958. Differences between smokers and non-smokers. Arch. Intern. Med. 101: 377-388.

Helman, R.M., Temko, M.H. and Fallon, H.J. 1969. Alcoholic hepatitis: Natural history and evaluation of therapy. Clin. Res. 17: 304 (Abst.).

Higgins, M.W., Kjelsberg, M., and Metzner, H. 1967. Characteristics of smokers and non-smokers in Tecumseh, Michigan. I. The distribution of smoking habits in persons and families and their relationships to social characteristics. Am. J. Epidemiol. 86: 45-59.

Hunter, J.M. 1976. Hypothermia and Wernicke's encephalopathy. Brit. Med. J. 2: 563-564.

Keys, A. 1945. Experimental studies on man with restricted intake of B vitamins. Am. J. Physiol. 144: 5-42.

Kowlessar, O.D. 1963. Diseases of the pancreas. IN *Cecil-Loeb's Textbook of Medicine*, Eds. Beeson, P.B. and McDermott, W. 11th Ed. W.B. Saunders Co.: Philadelphia and London. pp. 949-951.

Labadarios, D., Rossouw, J.E., McConnell, J.B., Davis, M. and William, R. 1977. Vitamin B_6 deficiency in chronic liver disease—evidence for increased degradation of pyridoxal-5'-phosphate. Gut 18: 23-27.

Le Gros Clark, F. 1968. Food habits as a practical nutrition problem. *World Review of Nutrition and Dietetics*, Vol. 9. Karger, Basel/New York. pp. 56-84.

Levy, J.L., Duga, J., Girgis, M. and Gordon, E.E. 1973. Ketoacidosis associated with alcoholism in non-diabetic subjects. Ann. Intern. Med. 78: 213-219.

Lischner, M.W., Alexander, J.F. and Galambos, J.T. 1971. Natural history of alcoholic hepatitis: I. The acute disease. Am. J. Dig. Dis. 16: 481-494.

McCarthy, R.G. 1951. *Facts About Alcohol.* Science Research Associates, Inc., Chicago.

Matarazzo, J.D. and Saslow, G. 1960. Psychological and related characteristics of smokers and non-smokers. Psychol. Bull. 57: 493-513.

Mellanby, E. 1920. Alcohol and alcoholic intoxication. Brit. J. Inebr. 17: 157-178.

Mello, N.K. 1972. Behavioral studies of alcoholism. IN *The Biology of Alcoholism.* II. Physiology and behavior. Kissin, B. and Begleiter, H., Eds. Plenum Press: New York, London. pp. 219-291.

Mello, N.K. and Mendelson, J.H. 1970. Experimentally induced intoxication in alcoholics: A comparison between programed and spontaneous drinking. J. Pharmacol. Exp. Ther. 173: 101-116.

Nilsson, E. and Westlin, N.E. 1970. Femur density in alcoholism and after gastrectomy. Calc. Tiss. Res. 10: 167-170.

Olsen, A.Y. 1950. A study of dietary factors, alcoholic consumption and laboratory findings in 100 patients with hepatic cirrhosis and 200 non-cirrhotic controls. Am. J. Med. Sci. 220: 477-484.

Palasciano, G., Tiscornia, O.M., Hagag, et al. 1974. Chronic alcoholism and endogenous cholecystokinine-pancreozymine (CCK-PZ). Biomed. 21:94-97.

Patek, A.J., Toth, I.G., Saunders, M.G., Castro, G.A.M. and Engel, J.J. 1975. Alcohol and dietary factors in cirrhosis. An epidemiological study of 304 alcoholic patients. Arch. Int. Med. 135: 1053-1057.

Pawan, L.S. 1974. Drugs and appetite. Proc. Nutr. Soc. 33: 239-244.

Perlow, W., Baraona, E. and Lieber, C.S. 1977. Symptomatic intestinal disaccharidase deficiency in alcoholics. Gastroenterology 72: 680-684.

Petersen, G. 1973. Alcoholism and ketoacidosis. Ann. Intern. Med. letter 78: 983.

Price, F.W. 1944. *A Textbook of the Practice of Medicine.* 6th Ed., Oxford Univ. Press: London. p. 582.

Roberts, D.M. 1972. Chronic gastritis, alcohol, an non-ulcer dyspepsia. Gut 13: 768-774.

Sauberlich, H.E. 1967. Biochemical alterations in thiamine deficiency—their interpretation. Am. J. Clin. Nutr. 20: 528-546.

Scott, C.C., Scott, W.W. and Luckhardt, A.B. 1938. Effect of alcohol on hunger sense. Am. J. Physiol. 123: 248-255.

Sedman, A.J., Wilkinson, P.K., Sakmar, E., Weidler, D.J. and Wagner, J.G. 1976. Food effects on absorption and metabolism of alcohol. Quart. J. Stud. Alc. 37: 1197-1213.

Smith, G.P. *et al.* 1974. Cholecystokinin and intestinal satiety in the rat. Fed. Proc. 33: 1146-1149.

Sullivan, J.F. and Burch, R.E. 1976. Potential role of zinc in liver disease. IN *Trace Elements in Human Health and Disease.* Vol. 1: Zinc and Copper. Eds. Prasad, A. and Oberleas, D. Academic Press: New York, San Francisco, London. p. 78.

Sullivan, J.F. and Lankford, H.G. 1965. Zinc metabolism and chronic alcoholism. Am. J. Clin. Nutr. 17: 57-63.

USDHEW Public Health Service. 1974. Alcohol and Health. Second Special Report to the U.S. Congress, Washington, D.C. M. Keller (Editor).

Vallee, B.L., Acker, W.E.C., Bartholomay, A.F. and Hoch, F.L. 1957. Zinc metabolism in hepatic dysfunction. II. Correlation of metabolic patterns with biochemical findings. New Eng. J. Med. 257: 1055-1065.

Victor, M. 1960. The role of nutrition in the alcoholic neurologic diseases. J. Clin. Invest. 39: 1037-1038. (Abst.).

Vilter, R.W. 1953. The effect of vitamin B_6 deficiency induced by desoxypyridoxine in human beings. J. Lab. Clin. Med. 42: 335-357.

Wilson, N.L. and Wilson, R.H.L. 1971. Dysnutrition and boredom. IN *Progress in Human Nutrition.* Ed. Margen, S. Vol. 1, AVI Publishing Co., Inc. Westport, Conn. pp. 111-117.

Wood, E.J. 1912. A treatise on pellagra for the general practitioner. Appleton: New York and London. pp. 144-150.

3

Alcohol Absorption and Metabolism

GASTROINTESTINAL ABSORPTION OF ALCOHOL

Though it is generally agreed that ethanol is absorbed by a process of simple diffusion across biological membranes in general, and across the gastrointestinal mucosa in particular, Kalant (1971) has pointed out that it is difficult to prove simple diffusion of ethanol in the human subject, because any attempt to do so would cause interference with normal physiological processes. This author also remarks that if it is to be proven that alcohol is absorbed by simple diffusion, then it should be possible to demonstrate that transfer follows Fick's Law. Fick's Law states that the amount of a substance diffusing across a unit area in unit time is equal to the concentration gradient across the surface in question multiplied by a diffusion coefficient, characteristic of the diffusing substance, and the membrane through which it is passing. Berggren and Goldberg (1940) conducted studies to test this hypothesis, and found that after closure of the pylorus with a ligature, absorption of ethanol from the cat's stomach followed predicted values, based on Fick's Law. Similarly, if ethanol was administered to human subjects, absorption from the stomach again followed this principle. Diffusion of ethanol through the stomach wall has been demonstrated at autopsy and in an *in vitro* experiment (Gifford and Turkel, 1956; Plueckhahn and Ballard, 1967; Karel and Fleisher, 1948).

Major factors which affect the absorption of ethanol from the gastrointestinal tract include concentration, the nature and surface area of the mucosa, the blood flow through the mucosal capillaries, the rate of stomach emptying, and the presence or absence of food in the gastrointestinal tract. Several older studies indicate a relationship between the amount of alcohol ingested and the concentration attained in the blood, urine, and alveolar air. Data obtained in these studies have been interpreted to show that the dilution in which the alcohol is drunk influences the concentration in the blood (Miles, 1922; and Schmidt, 1934).

Mellanby (1919), in studies on dogs, observed less intoxication following a specific amount of alcohol given as stout, as compared to that of dilute whiskey. By measuring the alcohol content of capillary blood samples, Mellanby found, in his experiments, that in spite of differences in the signs of intoxication exhibited by the dogs following whiskey or stout administration, the maximum concentrations of alcohol reached in the blood samples were similar. He also showed that the ingestion of a large amount of alcohol required more time for absorption than smaller amounts, as reflected by the time for alcohol to reach peak levels in the blood.

Mellanby's studies led him to the opinion that "the rate of oxidation (of alcohol) is constant throughout the whole period from the beginning of absorption to the end of oxidation and elimination, and that this is the case in spite of the fact that the amount of alcohol in the body is getting progressively less . . . Whatever the amount of alcohol in the body, the rate of oxidation is independent of the amount drunk." The rate of oxidation of alcohol, according to Mellanby, was approximately 0.148 gm alcohol/kg/hr. His conclusions were based on the rate of decrease of the concentration of alcohol in the blood for a period of six hours after administration of alcohol by the gastric route. Under these experimental conditions, the concentration of alcohol increased rapidly during the first hour and reached a maximum shortly thereafter. In the second hour, the level of alcohol in the blood remained practically constant (the Gréhant plateau). Then during the next four hours, concentrations of alcohol decreased slowly and uniformly, allowing Mellanby to make his conclusions about the constancy of alcohol oxidation. Criticizing Mellanby's conclusions, Haggard and Greenberg (1934) noted that in all of Mellanby's experiments, alcohol was administered by the gastric route, and that therefore it would be absorbed as well as oxidized during an undefined period following its administration. In other words, these authors are pointing out that it is unjustifiable to assume that alcohol absorption is complete at the time that the concentration of alcohol reaches its maximum in the blood, and therefore the declining concentration of alcohol expresses only oxidation and possibly excretion. It was shown by Haggard and Greenberg that when alcohol is administered by the enteral route, which in their experiments consisted in giving alcohol to dogs via the stomach, the amount of alcohol in the blood was shown to represent a balance between absorption and oxidation.

In a subsequent experiment, Harger and Hulpieu (1935) gave alcohol by stomach tube to dogs and at various intervals following the alcohol administration groups of the dogs were killed and the entire gastrointestinal tract was analyzed for its alcohol content. In another group of dogs which received the same dose of alcohol by intravenous administration in the form of a 12% saline solution, the intravenous administration took one hour and at the end of the second hour, these dogs were also killed and their gastrointestinal tracts analyzed for alcohol. The average concentrations of alcohol found in the gastrointestinal tracts of the dogs that had received alcohol by the intravenous route were subtracted from the corresponding figures of the dogs that got the alcohol by stomach tube to give an estimate of the concentration of unabsorbed alcohol. Complete absorption of the alcohol occurred in a period of approximately two hours. The results also indicated that alcohol is absorbed from the intestine as well as the stomach.

Völtz et al. (1912) were the first, in carrying out experiments on human subjects, to find out whether the observed protective effect of food ingestion against rapid intoxication was due to the influence of food on alcohol absorption. They gave moderate doses of alcohol to human subjects and showed that the alcohol content of urine was six times greater when the alcohol was taken on an empty stomach than when it was taken after food.

Mellanby (1920) had showed that the effect of food was to reduce concentrations of alcohol in the blood.

In a series of experiments, Widmarck (1933a, 1933b, 1935) showed that specific nutrients might depress blood alcohol levels in human subjects more than others. In particular, he found that amino acids lowered blood alcohol levels to a greater extent than fatty acids. However, his hypothesis that certain amino acids form complexes with ethanol in the gastrointestinal tract, thus preventing absorption, has not been substantiated (Haggard et al., 1940).

More recent authors (Miller and Sterling, 1966) have suggested that consumption of food may also increase the mean maximal rate of alcohol metabolism, although neither the work of these authors nor studies by Lundquist and Wolthers (1958), concerning effects of food on alcohol metabolism, indicates whether a concurrent administration of food with alcohol has an additional effect on alcohol metabolism as well as on the rate of alcohol absorption.

The lay observation that drinking milk before liquor reduces the risk of getting drunk was given scientific explanation by Miller et al. (1966). On each of two occasions, ten subjects, five men and five women, between the ages of 20 and 40, were given 25 ml of ethanol in the morning before breakfast. On the first occasion, the alcohol was given 90 minutes after the ingestion of a pint of water, and again 30 minutes after the ingestion of a further half-pint of water. On the second occasion, milk was substituted for the water. The authors comment that, because of the amount of alcohol given to all the subjects was the same, the effects on both blood alcohol concentration and on the degree of drunkenness would be roughly inversely proportional to body weight. When water was given, all the female subjects and three of the male subjects showed signs of intoxication. When the alcohol was taken with milk, intoxication was either lessened (3 subjects) or obviated (5 subjects). Blood alcohol levels were lower when the alcohol was given after milk rather than after water. The authors admit that their experimental protocol did not allow them to differentiate an effect of milk on alcohol absorption from an effect on alcohol metabolism.

It is interesting to see that Italian investigators have found it important to find out whether alcohol levels are different when food is administered with wine and whether blood alcohol levels are different when wine is taken in several small doses against the situation when it is taken all at once. Their interest arises from the fact that in Italy and in other wine drinking countries, it is customary to drink wine during meals and to refill wine glasses one or more times during the meal. Serianni et al. (1953) carried out several studies in which wine was given to healthy male medical students between the ages of 23 and 26. The wine given had an ethyl alcohol content of 11% by volume. Blood alcohol curves were studied after drinking the wine: a) in one dose in the fasting state; b) during the meal, i.e. when the subjects were halfway through the meal; and c) two hours, d) four hours, and e) six hours after the end of a meal. The meal, in each case, had a total energy value of 1898 kilocalories, and included spaghetti with tomato sauce, roast beef, fried potatoes, bread, and an apple.

Another series of experiments was carried out to evaluate differences between the ingestion of the same quantity of wine in one dose or several doses. In these studies, wine was given both in the fasting state and during the same standard meal in either three or six equal doses. When the wine was taken in three doses it was ingested every 10 minutes, and when in six doses, it was ingested every 5 minutes, to stimulate timing of meals and wine consumption during a standard meal lasting 30 minutes. The area under the blood alcohol curve was similar when the wine was given in the fasting state or six hours after the meal. When the wine was given with the meal, or two hours after the meal, the peak was reached earlier, and the area under the curve for blood alcohol values was reduced. When the wine was given four hours after the meal, the peak blood alcohol value was at 45 minutes after the start of wine drinking, which was similar to the time obtained with the wine given in the fasting state. However, in these circumstances, the area under the blood alcohol curve was intermediate between that when the wine was given in the fasting state and that when it was given with the meals or two hours after the meal. If the wine was given in the fasting state in three doses, the peak blood alcohol curve was reached later than when the same amount of wine was given on an empty stomach in a single dose. When the wine was given in the fasting state, in six doses, the peak was reached later than when it was given in the fasting state in three doses. When the wine was given during a meal in six doses, a peak was reached later than when it was given in six doses in the fasting state and also the area under the curve of blood alcohol levels was reduced. The authors conclude that when wine is given with or soon after meals, lower blood alcohol concentrations are found than when it is given in the fasting state and that, further, the effect of eating a large meal on blood alcohol concentrations lasts about four hours. The authors noted that the effects of meal eating are clearly seen, whether the wine is given in three or six doses during the meal.

Studies designed by Sedman *et al.* (1976) were carried out in order to make a statistical evaluation of the effects of various types of food on blood alcohol concentrations, and also to show whether, when food is given with alcohol, it has an effect on alcohol absorption or the rate of alcohol metabolism. Fourteen adult healthy men between the ages of 21 and 32 years were given three out of seven possible test meals which were randomly assigned. The treatments compared effects of alcohol consumed with fat, protein, or carbohydrate with alcohol taken in the fasting state. Treatments were administered at one-week intervals, and each treatment consisted in the administration of 45 ml of 95% diluted ethanol, with or without the above-mentioned foods or food substances. Venous blood samples were taken for blood alcohol determination using a gas chromatographic method. The area under the blood alcohol curve was significantly greater when alcohol was given in the fasting state than when the alcohol was given with fat, protein or soluble carbohydrate. A decrease in the area under the curve was found to be independent of the type of food administered. The time peak blood alcohol concentration and the peak alcohol concentration per se were found to be dependent on the type of food given. When alcohol was given with glucose, peak alcohol values were delayed, as contrasted with the time of occurrence of the peak with other treatments. The authors point out that the principle effect of food on the absorption of alcohol is likely to be a reduction in the rate of absorption. They cite earlier studies which indicated that different types of meals which delay gastric emptying induced the absorption rate for alcohol (Hunt, 1960; Hunt and Pathak, 1960; Hunt and MacDonald, 1954).

It is also important to note that Eisner and Berger (1971) found gastric emptying rate to be slowed significantly as the amount of glucose in a test load is increased.

It was later found by Sedman *et al.* (1976) that ingestion of a food containing any substance such as glucose, which slows gastric emptying, followed immediately by alcohol, resulted in a decreased area under the curve for blood alcohol values, decreased peak alcohol concentrations and an increased time for peak alcohol levels to occur. They further considered that, since food as such slows gastric emptying and therefore may decrease the rate of alcohol absorption, lower blood alcohol concentrations will result. This is explained by assuming that the relative efficiency of alcohol metabolism is greater at lower blood alcohol levels.

We may ask why there is a decreased rate of alcohol absorption under circumstances when gastric emptying time is slowed. Effects of food or food substances on gastric emptying are complex and the interactive effects of alcohol provide a challenge to the interpretation of any given situation of concomitant eating and drinking. Evidence that absorption of alcohol is more efficient from the duodenum and jejunum than from the stomach has been obtained both in animal and human studies (Payne *et al.*, 1966; Salvesen and Kolberg, 1958). Blood alcohol levels following oral test doses increase more rapidly and to a higher peak in patients who have had gastrectomies as compared to normal subjects (Elmslie *et al.*, 1965). Further, we may ask whether alcohol is absorbed better from the intestine than from the stomach. Differences in the rate of alcohol absorption from the stomach and small intestines undoubtedly reflect the principle set forth by Levine (1973), which states that "for any substance which can penetrate the gastrointestinal epithelium, in measureable amounts, the small intestine represents the area with the greatest capacity for absorption. This is true whether the molecule is relatively lipid soluble and not ionizable like alcohol, or is a weak electrolyte ..."

The older viewpoint was that gastric emptying could be regarded as exponential in form. Yet, when Hopkins (1966) examined the literature, he came to the conclusion that the pattern of gastric emptying in which "the square root of the volume of a meal remaining declines linearly with time, has been shown to account for the experimental results with less error."

A standard physiology text (Frolich, 1972) indicates that the rate of gastric emptying is directly proportional to the square root of the volume of the gastric contents. This concept does not fit the findings of recent studies.

Studies by Hedding *et al.* (1974) of normal subjects show that emptying of the aqueous phase of a meal can be approximated to a simple exponential process, but the solid phase empties at a constant rate. Emptying of the solid phase of the meal is substantially slower than that of the liquid phase.

Considering this newer information, it may be appreciated that the absorption of alcohol may be influenced directly by food composition as well as by the size of the meal. Further, Kalant (1971) has pointed out that the concentration of alcohol in the stomach can, in itself, alter the rate of gastric emptying. Larger doses of alcohol delay gastric emptying, probably because alcohol in high concentration paralyzes the smooth muscle of the stomach.

Several recent studies have shown that the composition of a meal as well as its size does, in fact, alter the rate and extent of alcohol absorption. Lynn *et al.* (1976) compared alcohol absorption in male subjects in the fasting state after a light breakfast, after a heavy breakfast, after a steak meal, one hour before and one hour after a heavy breakfast. The authors found that the rate and extent of alcohol absorption was decreased by food, but that reduction in the extent of alcohol absorption was more important than effects on the rate. In their studies, the largest reduction in the overall efficiency of alcohol absorption was found when alcohol was taken immediately after a heavy breakfast or a steak meal, and also when it was taken one hour after a heavy breakfast. Inhibition of alcohol absorption was less following a light meal, and was only slight in extent when alcohol was taken one hour before a meal.

Welling (1977) described studies carried out in his laboratory in which alcohol in low dosages (0.2 ml of 95% alcohol/kg body weight) was administered to six subjects either without food or immediately following high carbohydrate, high fat, or high protein meals. As in earlier studies, it was found that food per se reduced alcohol absorption but also that the reduction in alcohol absorption was greater when a carbohydrate meal was given.

It was shown by Levy and Jusko (1965) that increasing the viscosity of gastric contents by the addition of methyl cellulose decreases gastric absorption of ethanol in the rat. The mechanism proposed is that there is a slowing of diffusion of the alcohol molecules toward the absorptive surface of the gastric mucosa. In view of these findings, we are led to postulate that perhaps consumption of meals containing dietary fiber sources may also delay gastric emptying and reduced alcohol absorption.

Older studies suggest that alcohol from different alcoholic beverages is absorbed at different rates. From the time when modern methodologies for studying alcohol absorption were available, evidence was obtained that beer is absorbed more slowly than whiskey or brandy, that gin is absorbed more rapidly than whiskey, and that both gin and whiskey are absorbed more slowly than red wine. Kalant (1971) has suggested that ingredients of different beverages other than the alcohol may reduce gastric motility or perhaps blood flow, and it has futher been considered that perhaps either nutrients present in the alcoholic beverage, such as carbohydrate, or non-nutrient components may contribute to a reduction in gastric motility and thus to differences in alcohol absorption with various beverages (Haggard et al., 1938).

The need exists to re-examine absorption of different alcoholic beverages using up-to-date techniques and statistical analysis of data for comparison of blood alcohol curves.

ALCOHOL METABOLISM

Whereas Lundsgaard (1938) was the first to clearly demonstrate that the liver is the major organ for alcohol metabolism, more recent investigators have shown that alcohol may also be metabolized in other tissues, particularly in the kidney and in skeletal muscle (Larsen, 1963; Forsander et al. 1960). Myerson (1973), in reviewing the subject, has stated "As much as 20% of alcohol metabolism may occur in extrahepatic sites." Unchanged alcohol (ethanol) is excreted to a minor extent in the expired air, in the urine, and in the sweat, but more than 95% of ethanol taken into the body undergoes complete oxidation (Lundquist and Wolthers, 1958).

Ethanol oxidation is an effective source of energy because it is coupled with the synthesis of adenosine triphosphate (ATP). Three separate metabolic pathways exist for the oxidation of ethanol, which vary in biological importance (Lieber et al., 1975; Isselbacher and Greenberger, 1964). The first product in the metabolism of ethanol is always acetaldehyde. The main hepatic pathway for the formation of acetaldehyde involves the enzyme alcohol dehydrogenase (ADH) which is located in the cytosol of the hepatocytes. In the reaction, hydrogen is transferred from ethanol to the coenzyme nicotinamide adenine dinucleotide (NAD), which is converted to its reduced form.

$$CH_3CH_2OH + NAD^+ \xrightarrow[ADH]{} CH_3CHO + NADH + H^+$$

Accumulation of NADH in the liver leads to metabolic abnormalities.

Alcohol dehydrogenase is mainly localized in the liver, but it has also been found in extrahepatic tissues including the kidneys, gastrointestinal tract, lungs, testicular tissue and in the eye. Whereas in the liver, alcohol dehydrogenase is the enzyme which is responsible for the major production of acetaldehyde from ethanol under low or moderate levels of intake, it has other functions which have significance in the extrahepatic sites. In testicular tissue and in the retina, alcohol dehydrogenase acts in the conversion of retinol to retinal, thus playing a vital role in vitamin A-related functions pertaining to spermatogenesis and the visual process. With continued high intake of ethanol competition may exist between the function of alcohol dehydrogenase in the metabolism of ethanol and in vitamin A metabolism which may contribute to vitamin A deficiency in the alcoholic (Thompson, 1965).

An atypical form of the enzyme has been described which has an activity three to five times greater than that of the typical form, as well as having lower pH optimum. A series of isoenzymes of alcohol dehydrogenase have been isolated from the liver. Becker *et al.* (1974) indicated that when ethanol oxidation was catalyzed by alcohol dehydrogenase, there was evidence that this was the rate limiting step for the metabolic removal of ingested alcohol, although the velocity of the reaction may also depend upon the availability of NAD.

Recently Scholz and Nohl (1976) have performed further studies to determine whether the rate-controlling factor in ethanol metabolism is the activity of hepatic alcohol dehydrogenase. They note that this concept has been questioned because of observations that the rate of ethanol elimination varies with the metabolic state and can be stimulated by a number of different compounds including pyruvate and fructose. Using a liver perfusion technique, they were able to demonstrate that fructose stimulates ethanol oxidation in the rat. Their data led them to suggest that fructose stimulates ethanol oxidation indirectly, by increasing the energy consumption of the liver, because of an enhanced production of glucose from fructose. These findings provide evidence that maximal rates of NAD-dependent ethanol oxidation are determined by the activity of the respiratory chain, and hence on the energy requirements of the liver in a given metabolic state. Since a linear relationship was established between the extra NADH derived from ethanol oxidation, stimulated by fructose, and extra ATP utilized for fructose metabolism, it is these authors' hypothesis that the stimulation of ethanol oxidation by fructose is indirect and associated with the increased energy consumption of the liver. Actual steps in the metabolism of ethanol via the alcohol dehydrogenase-dependent pathway are as follows:

1. A molecule of alcohol dehydrogenase combines with a molecule of the coenzyme NAD in the oxidized state.

2. Ethanol is then bound to this complex and is oxidized such that the NAD accepts the liberated hydrogen.

3. Acetaldehyde so formed is released.

4. The reduced coenzyme NADH is detached from the alcohol dehydrogenase.

5. Alcohol dehydrogenase re-enters the same cycle (Becker *et al.*, 1974). The speed of alcohol metabolism by this pathway is dependent one rate of NADH reoxidation by the respiratory chain. Following the metabolism of ethanol to acetaldehyde by the alcohol dehydrogenase dependent path, further oxidation of acetaldehyde occurs with the production of acetic acid and the reduction of a further molecule of NAD:

acetaldehyde dehydrogenase

$$(CH_3 \cdot COH) + NAD + H_2O \rightarrow (CH_3 \cdot COOH) + NADH + H^+$$
Acetaldehyde   Acetic acid

This latter reaction is mainly mitochondrial. Krebs (1974) has emphasized that in the two reactions leading to the producton of acetic acid from ethanol, rather more than 60% of the reduced NAD is located in the cytoplasm and about 40% in the mitochondria. In order for the process of ethanol oxidation to continue, it is necessary for the NADH to be reconverted to NAD, which requires both molecular oxygen and intact mitochondrial electron transport. The capacity of this system is limited both by the capacity of electron carriers and also because oxidation must be coupled with phosphorylation. In the presence of ethanol, the rate of NADH production is larger than the capacity of the hepatocyte to remove it and this leads to further imbalance of the [NAD]/[NADH] ratio, such that here is an excess of NADH in the liver cytoplasm. It is known that acetyl coenzyme A (acetyl CoA) is formed from ethanol and presumably via acetate. Lieber (1975), however, has suggested that ethanol could be directly converted to acetyl CoA which could then yield acetate. Blood acetate has been shown to increase after ethanol administration (Crouse *et al.*, 1968).

Two alcohol-dehydrogenase-independent systems of alcohol metabolism in the liver have been identified. At low concentrations, alcohol is mainly oxidized through the alcohol dehydrogenase system which, as already described, is limited by the supply by NAD^+ or by the rate at which NADH produced in the reaction can be reoxidized (Videla and Israel, 1970; Hillboom, 1971). At higher concentrations of alcohol, oxidation is also carried out via a catalase-dependent reaction, which is limited by the rate of hydrogen peroxide generation. The reaction is as follows:

$$CH_3CH_2OH + H_2O_2 \xrightarrow[\text{catalase}]{} CH_3CHO + 2H_2O$$

Although it has been intimated by several investigators (Thurman, 1973; Oshino et al., 1973) that at higher concentrations of alcohol the oxidation is via the catalase pathway, Lieber et al. (1975) calculated that less than 2% of ethanol ingested is oxidized by this mechanism.

Observations in the rat, that ethanol feeding causes a proliferation of smooth endoplasmic reticulum in hepatocytes similar to that seen after the administration of other foreign compounds, which are metabolized by the mixed function oxidase system, led to investigation of whether alcohol could be metabolized by this system (Iseri et al., 1964; Iseri et al., 1966).

A mixed function oxidizing system capable of metabolizing ethanol was described by Orme et al. in 1965, and confirmed by Lieber and DeCarli (1968; 1970). Evidence suggests that the mixed function oxidase system is important in the metabolism of ethanol when high concentrations are present (Lieber et al., 1975). The suggestion that 20% of alcohol metabolism is via the mixed function oxidase system has been made by Myerson (1973). This system is NADPH-dependent as represented in the following equation:

$$CH_3CH_2OH + NADPH + H^+ + O_2 \xrightarrow[\text{MFOS}]{} CH_3CHO + NADP + H_2O$$

THE RELATIONSHIP BETWEEN ALCOHOL METABOLISM AND LIVER DAMAGE

Increases in the rate of alcohol metabolism have been reported among recent drinking alcoholics, particularly those who are chronic drinkers, and also in alcohol-treated rats (Kater et al. 1969; Ugarte et al. 1972; Videla and Israel, 1970). Ugarte et al. (1977) studied the rate of ethanol metabolism in alcoholics with normal livers; alcoholics with fatty livers without necrosis; alcoholics with liver necrosis and severe steatosis as well as fibrosis, and those with mild fibrosis not associated with other lesions. Control subjects were healthy males who were occasional or moderate drinkers with an alcohol intake of less than 50 g/day. The alcoholic patients were studied after a variable period of abstinence of between 9 and 25 days. All subjects were given one gram of alcohol/kg body weight and 250 ml of saline over a period of 20 minutes, one hour after a breakfast meal consisting in a cup of coffee with milk and sugar, and 100 g of white bread. The alcohol was given by the intravenous route, and venous blood samples were obtained at 30 min., 60 min., 90 min., 120 min. and 150 min. after the completion of the infusion. Blood ethanol values were determined in all these samples. Ethanol metabolism was calculated according to the method of Widmarck (1933a), by expressing blood alcohol clearance in mg/kg body weight/hr. Liver biopsies, obtained 40 to 74 hrs. before the alcohol infusion, allowed the identification of steatosis, alcohol hepatitis and fibrosis. With each diagnosis, the degree of liver damage was graded according to a pre-determined numerical system. It was found that the rate of ethanol metabolism was increased in patients with liver disease as compared to control subjects and that the patients with severe liver disease, including those with necrosis or necrosis with cirrhosis had a rate of ethanol metabolism exceeding the other groups.

Objections that may be raised with respect to the interpretation of this study are the variable period of abstinence between groups and between subjects. Further, there is the confusing fact that 43 of the alcoholic cases, who presented with mild alcohol withdrawal syndromes, received meprobamate at a dose of 800 mg/day, which could alter the rate of metabolism. (This drug was apparently stopped at least 5 days before the IV alcohol testing.)

A further difficulty arises in interpreting the studies by Ugarte et al. (1977), in that most authors have found a decrease in alcohol dehydrogenase activity in the livers of patients with steatosis or cirrhosis (von Wartburg, 1971). In the 1977 review of the effects of alcohol by von Wartburg, it is made clear that large differences may exist in the rate of alcohol metabolism between individuals. These differences are dependent upon genetic variability in the alcohol dehydrogenase enzyme and on whether an "atypical enzyme" is present. A more plausible interpretation of the work by Ugarte et al. is that in the alcoholic subject, the degree of liver damage is related to the period of alcoholism. It was suggested by Lieber et al. in 1975 that ethanol administration or chronic intake does result in an increased rate of metabolism (we suggest that induced changes in the rate of ethanol metabolism are perhaps via the mixed function oxidase system).

METABOLIC AND NUTRITIONAL VARIABLES IN ALCOHOLIC LIVER DISEASE

Ever since it was established that the whole spectrum of alcoholic liver disease, from steatosis to hepatitis, and from hepatitis to cirrhosis, can be produced in rats, in subhuman primates, and probably in human subjects by alcohol consumption, and independently of a grossly deficient diet, the question has arisen as to the mechanism whereby alcohol or its metabolites induce the liver damage (Iseri *et al.*, 1966; Rubin *et al.*, 1970; Lieber *et al.*, 1965; Rubin and Lieber, 1967; 1968; 1974; Lieber and Rubin, 1968).

According to Stege *et al.* (1976), acetaldehyde derived from ethanol oxidation may cause lipid peroxidative trauma to the liver mitochondria. Such mitochondrial injury is believed by these authors to impair acetaldehyde metabolism, such that further peroxidative injury takes place. It is proposed that with chronic alcoholism, progressive liver disease may result from this cycle of events.

Our present concept of the biochemical sequence of events in the development of a fatty liver in alcoholics was first suggested by Krebs (1968; 1974). In a 1968 study, Krebs found a six-fold increase in the concentration of alpha-glycerophosphate in perfused livers after ethanol dosing. He pointed out that in the synthesis of triglyceride, "alpha-glycerophosphate reacts with two molecules of the coenzyme A ester of fatty acids to form a diglyceride phosphate. This is followed by the release of phosphate and a reaction of the diglyceride so formed with another coenzyme A ester of fatty acid to produce a triglyceride." The increased relative concentrations of $NADH_2$ favor production of alpha-glycerophosphate.

A very interesting study by Baker *et al.* (1973) indicates that, at least in the rat, administration of niacin (nicotinic acid) can prevent the accumulation of nonesterified fatty acid, total fat and neutral fat in the liver of animals who have been fed ethanol. Since blood ethanol levels remain elevated after this treatment, the authors postulated that perhaps niacin acted by blocking ethanol oxidation through an inhibition of alcohol dehydrogenase. In these investigations, the rats received pharmacologic doses of niacin which are known in human subjects as well as in experimental animals to reduce blood levels of circulating lipids.

A question which has been much disputed is the nature of alcoholic cirrhosis. This disease commonly occurs as a sequel of alcoholic hepatitis, although there is considerable documentation to suggest that cirrhosis can develop insidiously without overt clinical signs of hepatitis (Popper, 1976).

The fact that alcoholic cirrhosis can be induced in subhuman primates by prolonged ethanol feeding, with maintenance of the animals on an "adequate diet" does not mean that there is not a nutritional component in the development of cirrhosis. Alcoholic liver disease is similar to alcoholic disease of other tissues in that in its chronic form, the cells of the liver are unable to utilize nutrients to normal capacity. The demonstration that methotrexate, a folacin antagonist, will frequently induce liver fibrosis or cirrhosis in alcoholics, prompts the suggestion that investigation should be carried out to examine relationships between the development of cirrhosis and the presence of folacin deficiency.

ALCOHOL INDUCED METABOLIC DISORDERS — THEIR NUTRITIONAL COMPONENT

In acute or chronic alcohol abuse, the metabolic functions of the liver are disturbed. Functions of the liver include synthesis, interconversion, metabolism, transport, storage, and excretion of nutrients as well as endogeneous compounds including hormones, pyrroles, and purines. It is therefore not surprising that, with ethanolic liver damage, nutritional as well as multiple metabolic errors may arise. Whether or not

METABOLIC FUNCTIONS OF THE LIVER

Function	Product
Synthesis	Plasma proteins Urea Glycogen Triglyceride Free fatty acid Cholesterol Heme
Regulation	Glucose Hormone Pyrrole Nutrient (levels in plasma)
Metabolism/clearance	Monosaccharides Lactate Cholesterol Free fatty acids Amino acids Hormones
Storage	Glycogen Vitamins - water and fat soluble Iron

These metabolic functions are particularly vulnerable with respect to effects of ethanol.

particular metabolic aberrations occur in individuals depends not only on their genetic makeup, but also is critically dependent on their nutrient intake at the time of alcohol abuse, on age, physiological status, stress, previous history of liver disease, intake of or exposure to toxic environmental chemicals including drugs and treatment of the alcoholic episode.

GLUCONEOGENESIS AND ALCOHOLIC HYPOGLYCEMIA

Severe, profound or fatal hypoglycemia may occur after episodes of binge drinking, particularly when the alcoholic excess is associated with zero food intake. Vulnerable people include children and those with preexisting alcoholic liver disease. Ingestion of high levels of alcohol inhibits gluconeogenesis. Inhibition of the key enzyme in gluconeogenesis, pyruvate carboxylase, by the increased liver cell NADH to NAD ratio is believed to be the basic mechanism in the development of the impairment in gluconeogenesis. Furthermore, it is known that liver glycogen can be depleted by a period of fasting not in excess of 72 hours and in certain instances after a shorter period. A combination of glycogen depletion and adequate gluconeogenesis largely accounts for the observed hypoglycemia. In addition, it is known that oxidation of galactose, which is also a hepatic function, is inhibited by alcohol (Isselbacher, 1977).

It was emphasized by Madison (1968) that alcohol-induced hypoglycemia not only occurs in alcoholics who are malnourished, but also in binge drinkers when no food is taken during the binge, and in young children who may drink alcohol accidentally. The risk of this potentially fatal condition for children has also been recognized and reported by other authors (Golding, 1970; Heggarty, 1970). The signs and symptoms of alcoholic hypoglycemia are similar to those of diabetic hypoglycemia and include weakness, tremulousness, mental confusion, bizarre behavior, incoherent speech, sweating, tachycardia, and if not promptly treated, hypoglycemic coma, which will respond to intravenous administration of glucose.

Arky *et al.* (1968) reported on five patients with insulin-dependent diabetes who were also alcoholics and who were hospitalized with hypoglycemia after an alcohol binge. Of these patients, two died without coming out of hypoglycemic coma and those who survived had severe neurological damage.

ALCOHOLIC HYPERURICEMIA AND GOUT

Hyperuricemia has been reported both in non alcoholics who are acutely inebriated, and also in chronic alcoholics after the intake of alcohol (Lieber *et al.*, 1962a). Serum lactate levels are increased, and there is a diminished renal output of uric acid (Isselbacher and Greenberger, 1964). As Lieber and his colleagues have demonstrated (1962b), it is the increased NADH/NAD intracellular ratio which leads to an increased lactate/pyruvate ratio, which in turn results in hyperlactacidemia. It is the hyperlactacidemia which reduces the kidneys' capacity to excrete uric acid, and hence, causes the development of hyperuricemia.

Historical accounts as well as modern clinical observations have indicated that attacks of gout may be precipitated by alcohol binges, particularly when these are accompanied by food restriction. Effects of fasting, alcohol ingestion and combinations of these on serum uric acid levels and attacks of acute gout were studied by MacLachlan and Rodnan (1967). Subjects in the study were nine patients with gout and two normouricemic controls. Eight of the gouty patients were males, as well as both of the control patients. Elevated serum urate levels were found in the patients after one and two days fasts and the elevated levels in serum urate were associated with a decreased urinary excretion of uric acid which the investigators assumed to be the result of decreased tubular secretion of urate. Administration of moderate doses of alcohol (68-100 gms) in the form of rye whiskey or beer produced only minor changes in serum urate and urinary uric acid excretion. Larger doses of alcohol given with food were followed by significant increases in serum uric acid and diminution in urinary uric acid output. These changes in uric acid levels of blood and urine were associated with increased blood lactate concentrations. Smaller doses of alcohol did not affect, or only slightly affected, the serum urate levels when taken with food. Increases in serum urate levels with low dose alcohol were greater than serum urate changes found with fasting alone. It is suggested that the combination of alcohol intake and fasting potentiate one another in their effects on uric acid metabolism. Eight of the nine patients who were included in the study had one or more attacks of acute gout during these investigations. It was observed that these gouty attacks occurred both with sudden increases in serum urate levels associated with fasting, or with similar rises in serum urate concentrations occurring when fasting was associated with alcohol intake. Physicians are cautioned to suggest to the patients with gout that both fasting and imbibing alcoholic beverages excessively can produce an attack. It is noted that gouty patients who enjoy alcohol do not deliberately abstain from food, but that a drinking binge may nevertheless continue for a period of time without food being taken, and that this combination of circumstances induces the gouty attack. Three possible explanations are offered by these authors for the increase in serum uric acid levels in their subjects which occurred either during periods of fasting or when alcohol was given in the fasting state. Reference is made to the studies of Lieber *et al.* (1962) showing that increases in blood lactate levels produced during alcohol oxidation may lead to lowered urinary uric acid excretion and hence elevation in serum urate.

In 1923, Gibson and Doisy observed that hyperlactacidemia, artificially produced in normal subjects by administration of ten to fourteen grams of sodium lactate, was followed by a decreased renal excretion of uric acid.

It has been shown, on the other hand, in fasting subjects and in those on high fat diets, that elevation of serum uric acid levels associated with decreased urinary uric acid excretion is associated with elevation in aceto acids in the blood including beta-hydroxybutyric acid and acetoacetic acid (Scott *et al.*, 1964; Lecocq and McPhaul, 1965).

Goldfinger *et al.* (1965) showed that renal retention of uric acid could be induced by infusion of beta-hydroxybutyrate and acetoacetate.

When the gouty patients investigated by MacLachlan and Rodnan (1967) were fasted for two days, there was a uniform rise in serum urate levels which quickly reverted to normal by feeding. These changes in serum urate were not accompanied by significant changes in blood lactate levels but beta-hydroxybutyrate serum values rose to levels which were sufficient to inhibit the urinary excretion of uric acid. Under the conditions of fasting and alcohol intake, the same patients showed increases in serum lactate levels and also increases in serum beta-hydroxybutyrate. It was suggested by these authors that higher levels of blood lactate of the beta-hydroxybutyrate which were found in the patients after fasting and alcohol ingestion induced a greater inhibition of the renal excretion of uric acid than did fasting alone.

Elevation in serum uric acid values and reduction in urinary urate excretion levels occurred not only in gouty patients but also in normal subjects following fasting and fasting with intake of alcoholic beverages. Seegmiller (1974) lists many chemical substances causing an inhibition of uric acid excretion. Among these are lactic acid, beta-hydroxybutyric acid, branch chain keto acids, and catecholamines. He further associates hyperuricemia with renal retention of uric acid with starvation, diabetic ketoacidosis and alcohol ingestion.

ALCOHOL - INDUCED PORPHYRIA

Disorders of pyrrole metabolism collectively known as the porphyrias have, in the past, been divided into the hepatic and erythropoietic forms; this designation suggesting the site of abnormal pyrrole synthesis. Although in view of recent studies, subdivision of porphyrias into hepatic and erythropoietic has been questioned, it is still true that those porphyrias previously considered as hepatic are the metabolic diseases within this group which are more commonly induced by environmental chemicals. In human subjects, the substances which are known to have a capacity for inducing acquired hepatic porphyrias, or of producing acute attacks of genetically determined porphyrias, are alcohol, estrogens, and halogenated aromatic compounds. Our present concern is with the relationship of ethanol to the development of acquired symptomatic porphyria (porphyria cutanea tarda) and inherited variegate porphyria. These porphyrias are characterized by an increased synthesis or activity of the enzyme delta aminolevulinic acid synthetase, which is the rate limiting enzyme in heme synthesis. Increased activity of this enzyme occurs because of metabolic blocks or partial blocks in the heme-biosynthetic pathway; these blocks being unique for each of the porphyrias. End product repression of heme synthesis normally occurs.

Etiological relationships between the development of porphyria cutanea tarda and alcohol abuse are supported by the disease history, clinical findings and organ pathology. Hepatic disease is common in patients with porphyria cutanea tarda. The liver, as well as other tissues, exhibits siderosis (excessive deposition of iron). The disease is biochemically characterized by moderate increases in the activity of delta aminolevulinic acid synthetase, increased production of uroporphyrin and coproporphyrin, and deposition of these porphyrins in the tissues. Liver biopsy specimens from patients with this disease show a variety of histological abnormalities (Eales, 1963; Bogorad, 1963; DeMatteis, 1967; Uys and Eales, 1963; Lundvall et al., 1970; Timme, 1971; Waldo and Tobias, 1973; Timme et al., 1974; Turnbull, 1971).

The high prevalence of alcohol abuse among patients with porphyria cutanea tarda has been confirmed by many investigators; however, Bloom (1976) pointed out that the hepatic changes found in these patients with this disease are not identical with those seen in alcoholics. It was his opinion that patients with porphyria cutanea tarda are predisposed to the effects of alcohol. He also suggested that increased hepatic production of uroporphyrin may in itself be hepatotoxic.

Studies by Benedetto et al. (1978) indicate that porphyria cutanea tarda is a familial disease inherited as an autosomal doinant trait and characterized by decreased erythrocyte and hepatic uroporphyrinogen decarboxylase activity. Clinical expression may be secondary to alcoholism and hepatic siderosis which further reduces hepatic activity of uroporphyrinogen decarboxylase.

Attacks of acute intermittent porphyria are precipitated by fasting. Similar phenomena have been observed in experimental rats made porphyric by administration of the drug, allylisopropylacetamide (Rose *et al.*, 1961; Welland *et al.*, 1964). In discussing a young patient whose acute intermittent porphyria was precipitated by an eight day therapeutic fast for weight reduction, Knudsen (1967) comments that fasting produces increases in a number of hepatic enzymes including delta aminolevulinic acid synthetase, and that this may be the explanation for the "starvation porphyric."

The fact that alcohol excess has also been reported as a factor responsible for the induction of attacks of acute intermittent porphyria has been interpreted by some to indicate an association rather than a causal relationship. Under conditions of alcohol abuse, there may be concomitant abstention from food, and it is actually the fasting state which precipitates attacks of the disease (Goldberg and Rimington, 1962; Eales, 1971). The present author agrees with the conclusions of Tschudy (1975), that decreased food intake, in periods of alcoholic excess, precipitate and/or maintain attacks on acute intermittent porphyria.

Haberman *et al.* (1975) noted a strong resemblance between porphyria cutanea tarda developing following intake of estrogens and the same disease occurring in alcoholics. Management of such cases would depend upon the duration of the disease. In early cases, discontinuation of the estrogens or alcohol abstention associated with an adequate diet will cause a remission. In established cases of porphyria cutanea tarda, phlebotomy is the treatment of choice, causing mobilization of the iron which is deposited in the hepatocytes, perhaps thereby interfering with the normal heme synthesis.

ZIEVE'S HEMOLYTIC ANEMIA AND ALCOHOLIC HYPERLIPEMIA

It was in 1958 that Zieve described 20 alcoholic patients who exhibited a syndrome of liver disease, hyperlipemia and transient hemolytic anemia. The suggestion was made that the combination of these findings constituted a new syndrome. Since that time, other investigators have reported similar patients and in addition incomplete forms of the syndrome have been observed (Fukuda, 1964; Haber, 1961; Smith *et al.*, 1964; Ström, 1963; Whitcomb and Job, 1960;

Dalmau-ciria, 1962; Petite, 1964; Zieve and Hill, 1959; 1961).

Viewpoints have differed as to whether there is an etiological relationship between hyperlipemia and hemolytic anemia in alcoholics. Zieve (1958) and Kessel (1962) suggested that hemolysis in hyperlipemic alcoholic patients with liver disease could be caused by the presence of small amounts of an abnormal circulating lipid.

Blass and Dean (1966) described an alcoholic patient with hyperlipemic jaundice, hemolytic anemia and pancreatitis. Examination of this patient's plasma and a plasma lipid extract showed no difference in hemolytic activity as compared with similar extracts from a normal subject. This patient exhibited increased plasma lysolecithin levels which had been suggested by Zieve to be a possible cause of hemolytic anemia, since lysolecithin does cause hemolysis *in vitro*. Alcoholic patients, however, have been described with normal serum lysolecithin levels but presenting with liver disease, hyperlipemia and hemolytic anemia (Robinson, 1961; Collier, 1952).

Several different types of hemolytic anemia have been described in alcoholic patients, particularly those with advanced liver disease. Eichner (1973), who has classified these anemias and discussed whether Zieve's syndrome is, in fact, a single clinical entity, emphasizes that there is no substantive evidence that hyperlipemia is, in fact, directly and causally related to hemolytic anemia.

While the mechanism for the development of Zieve's syndrome is not well understood, Lieber (1975) has suggested that there may be an extra corpuscular hemolytic factor as well as a change in the lipid composition of the red cell membrane (Balcerzak *et al.*, 1968; Powell *et al.*, 1972; Westerman *et al.*, 1968).

In the rat, fatty liver hyperlipemia and changes in the erythrocyte can be induced by administration of alcohol (Baraona and Lieber, 1969).

While it seems likely that not all the cases previously accepted as Zieve's syndrome can be accepted as being of one etiology, explanations have been offered for the association of hemolytic anemia and hyperlipemia in alcoholic patients. Eichner and Hillman (1971) suggested that some cases of so-called Zieve's syndrome may represent the stage of resolution of sideroblastic and megaloblastic anemia due respectively to vitamin B_6 and folacin deficiency in alcoholics. After alcohol ingestion is discontinued in such patients and a normal diet instituted, patients may exhibit a normoblastic erythroid hyperplasia and high reticulocyte count, suggestive of a hemolytic process. Clinicians are cautioned by these authors that these are not signs of a hemolytic process, and that a true hemolytic anemia should not be diagnosed unless hematologic studies show a reduced red cell life span.

Hemolytic anemia may be associated with acute pancreatitis, whether or not hyperlipemia is also present. Jacob and Amsden (1971) described a 47-year old alcoholic man who presented with acute pancreatitis, severe metabolic acidosis and a hemolytic anemia associated with red cell rigidity. He was found to have an extreme hypophosphatemia with a serum phosphorus of less than 0.1 mg/100ml. During the time that he was hypophosphatemic, red cell survival was greatly shortened, and red cell ATP levels were less than 15% of the normal values. It is suggested that the severe hypophosphatemia led to a hemolytic anemia because a certain minimal level of red cell ATP is required for the normal plasticity of the red cell, and if this level is not maintained, red cell integrity is lost.

A question that may be asked is whether the biochemical changes associated with acute pancreatitis could cause hemolytic anemia. In dogs, given large quantities of pancreatitic enzymes intravenously, hemolytic anemia may ensue (Walters and Owen, 1963). However, the association of pancreatitis and hemolytic anemia is rare in human subjects. It seems that Zieve's syndrome is confusing if its components are considered as being causally related. However, this does not mean that the components of the syndrome are not a clearcut complex. Hypertriglyceridemia is common in alcoholic subjects with liver disease. Isselbacher and Greenberger (1964) emphasized that hypertriglyceridemia and pancreatitis are also frequently found to co-exist in alcoholics.

Pancreatitis may be associated with the other signs of Zieve's syndrome and may, by inducing phosphate depletion, cause hemolytic anemia. However, hypertriglyceridemia does not in itself cause hemolytic anemia (Cooper and Shattil, 1971).

Pancreatitis in alcoholics tends to occur in those patients whose diet is rich in fat and animal protein, and in experimental dogs and rats given alcohol, pancreatitis will develop if these animals are also maintained on a similar diet (Sarles, 1977).

The interpretation of Zieve's syndrome has been well-stated by Jones (1969). He concludes "in some cases of alcoholic hyperlipemia with documented hemolysis, the hemolysis persisted after the hyperlipemia had cleared and the hemolysis cannot have been due to the hyperlipemia per se. Hyperlipemia can be induced by alcohol without affecting the red blood cell survival time, and clinical cases of alcoholic hyperlipemia occur without anemia. Therefore, although anemia may certainly accompany alcoholic hyperlipemia and fatty liver, in many cases it does not seem to be pathogenetically related to the hyperlipemia itself."

While there is no evidence that dietary aberrations in the alcoholic are directly responsible for alcoholic hyperlipemia, alcoholic liver disease or hemolytic anemia, various metabolic defects pertaining to the disposition of nutrients can account for association of hemolytic disease or apparent hemolytic disease and hyperlipemia in alcoholics, particularly those with liver disease.

METABOLIC AND NUTRITIONAL EFFECTS OF ALCOHOL WITHDRAWAL

Mild reactions to alcohol withdrawal are associated with tremulousness, insomnia, irritability and anorexia. Anxiety and tension headache, often incorrectly diagnosed as migraine, may be present. Among our patients who are frequent binge drinkers, alcohol withdrawal is often followed by an intense craving for salt or, less commonly, sugar. Severe acute alcohol withdrawal symptoms include tremulousness, hallucinations of a visual or auditory type, seizures and a confusional state. Since alcohol withdrawal is often determined by hospitalization for alcohol related diseases, acute infection or injury, the signs of withdrawal are often complicated by these other problems. The effect of these interventive health problems, requiring acute care, on the overall treatment of alcohol withdrawal has been discussed by Sellers and Kalant (1976).

In the present context, we have to ask two questions: firstly, whether any of the signs of alcohol withdrawal are influenced by recent diet and secondly, whether the clinical features can be explained by nutrient deficiency consequent on alcohol intoxication or abuse. In reports by Mendelson (1964) and Mello (1972), it has been emphasized that alcohol withdrawal signs and symptoms can occur "in healthy, well nourished alcoholics" and can be explained as being due to withdrawal of ethanol in an alcohol dependent person.

The finding by Leevy et al. (1965), that patients exhibiting delirium tremens, the most severe form of withdrawal syndrome, had low circulating vitamin levels may be variously interpreted.

Despite "adequate diets," alcoholics are more liable to develop hypovitaminemia because of malabsorption, hyperexcretion or impaired utilization of these micronutrients. Furthermore, at the point at which an alcoholic is encouraged to enter a detoxication unit, or arrives in a hospital after an accident, or is jailed for an alcohol-related misdemeanor, an alcoholic spree may have directly preceded the event during which time food may have been withheld. Vitamin or mineral levels in the blood may not accurately reflect a state of chronic malnutrition under these circumstances. A point which has been raised by Feuerlein (1977) is whether some of the signs previously connected with the alcohol withdrawal syndrome including vomiting and perhaps loss of appetite are not actually signs of persistent intoxication.

Delirium tremens may actually occur while alcohol ingestion is continued, though change in the level of alcohol intake, usually by reduction but sometimes by increase, usually precedes onset of symptoms. In this condition, hallucinations are very prominant and vivid, and autonomic system disorders occur with tachycardia, pyrexia and sweating. In view of these absolute diagnostic criteria for delirium tremens, many authors have defended its separate recognition from the more usual alcohol withdrawal syndrome (Feuerlein, 1977). Leevy et al. (1969) mentioned that administration of B vitamins including thiamin, niacin and pyridoxine may hasten the resolution of the mental and physical aberrations which occur in delirium tremens in some patients.

Hypomagnesemia has been found in alcoholics during periods of withdrawal, and more particularly during delirium tremens. A causal relationship between the magnesium depletion and the psychiatric manifestations of delirium tremens was suggested by Flink et al. (1954).

Magnesium deficiency is associated with tremor, bizarre movements, convulsions and delirium (Flink et al., 1957). On the basis of their own studies and a literature review, Flink et al. (1969) considered that magnesium depletion explains the signs and symptoms of delirium tremens. They justified this conclusion with the following observations:

"1. Significant magnesiopenia.
2. The similarity of the symptoms and signs to that of non-alcoholic patients with magnesium deficiency.
3. A significant negative magnesium balance in alcoholics.
4. Demonstrated decrease in exchangeable magnesium in alcoholic patients.
5. A significant decrease in muscle magnesium concentration.
6. A significant decrease in red cell magnesium.
7. A favorable response of alcoholics with delirium tremens to treatment with magnesium salts."

They claim that the whole spectrum of clinical features of delirium tremens has been seen in non-alcoholic patients who have magnesium depletion. Nevertheless, the identity of magnesium deficiency and delirium tremens is not confirmed. Wolfe and Victor (1969) found that the magnesium level in the serum may actually be increased at the onset of the delirium tremens.

Whether or not magnesium deficiency is the cause of withdrawal symptoms, and particularly the cause of symptoms of delirium tremens, remains in debate. However, there is a definite association between magnesium deficiency and alcohol abuse. Flink (1971) has enumerated causes of magnesium deficiency in alcoholics and these include decrease in food intake, particularly during the withdrawal period, inadequate magnesium intake, ketosis resulting both from the semi-starvation and from the metabolic effects of ethanol causing a negative magnesium balance, and excessive urinary excretion of magnesium due to the toxic effect of ethanol in the kidney. It was Flink's observation that magnesium repletion in non-alcoholic deficiency induces a prompt response, whereas if magnesium is given in the treatment of delirium tremens, response may be delayed for 48 to 72 hours. Facts to remember are that magnesium deficiency in itself causes severe electrolyte imbalance such that hypomagnesemia is associated with hypocalcemia and hypokalemia. Neurological signs in withdrawal syndromes and in delirium tremens would appear to be compounded of hypomagnesemia, co-existing electrolyte imbalance, respiratory alkalosis, and perhaps interference by alcohol with neural function (Feuerlein, 1977).

NUTRIENT TOXICITY IN HEPATOCELLULAR FAILURE AND HEPATIC ENCEPHALOPATHY

Hepatic encephalopathy is the neurological syndrome associated with hepatic failure. Signs include intermittent somnolence, reversal of day-to-night sleep patterns, bizarre behavior, episodes of stupor, and coma. A flapping tremor of the outstretched arms and hands (asterixis) is diagnostic. Without effective treatment this condition is fatal. In alcoholics with severe hepatitis or more commonly in those with Laennec's cirrhosis, hepatic encephalopathy may be recurrent or terminal. It is most likely to occur in alcoholics with cirrhosis who have undergone porto-caval shunts to overcome complications associated with portal hypertension. Sherlock (1963) comments that hepatic encephalopathy with coma can be precipitated by a high intake of protein, by administration of ammonium chloride, ingestion of a higher dose of methionine, by electrolyte imbalance complicating paracentesis to relieve ascites, or by administration of oral diuretics.

Present concepts of the etiology of hepatic encephalopathy have been summarized by Maddrey and Weber (1975) in a statement that the altered cerebral metabolism is due to "various metabolic products of gut origin normally cleared from portal vein blood by the intact liver."

Events preceding hepatic encephalopathy in the alcoholic include shunting of the portal blood into the systemic circulation and nitrogen overload. Actual precipitating factors include gastrointestinal hemorrhage which introduces large amounts of blood proteins into the gastrointestinal tract; high intake of dietary protein with or without amino acid supplements such as methionine, the catabolic state associated with infections, and constipation which causes excessive microbial metabolism of nitrogenous waste in the colon. When upper gastrointestinal hemorrhage precedes hepatic failure and encephalopathy, causes include bleeding esophageal varices and very commonly acute mucosal ulcers caused by ingestion of aspirin or other anti-inflammatory drugs (Franco et al., 1977).

Ammonia is believed to be the cerebral toxin responsible for hepatic encephalopathy. However, whether ammonia is the only cerebral toxin responsible for the cerebral manifestations of hepatic failure is still unclear. In the colon, ammonia is produced through microbial action on intraluminal nitrogenous substrates. These nitrogenous substrates include undigested protein when maldigestion is present, blood, secreted plasma proteins, urea and nitrogen derived from the intestinal microflora. In patients with cirrhosis, the mechanism for ammonia removal is inadequate and ammonia may reach the brain either recycled by the enterohepatic circulation or by passing directly into systemic circulation. It has been found that the ammonia load is increased by potassium depletion which may follow administration of diuretics as well as by the presence of bacteria in the small intestine. Strong support for the etiological role of ammonia in the production of hepatic encephalopathy has come from clinical experience of the use of nonabsorbable antibiotics such as neomycin which, by reducing the bacteria of microflora of the intestine, effectively decrease ammonia production and at the same time, reverse hepatic encephalopathy (Faloon, 1972).

A suggestion has been made that since elevated serum methionine levels are frequently found in patients with hepatic encephalopathy, this amino acid or its degradation products may be associated with the disorder. If hepatic encephalopathy is actually induced by the administration of methionine, the state can be reversed by giving antibiotics and it has been suggested that the toxic degradation products could either be methylmercaptan and dimethylsulfide, or that these products may serve as sources of ammonia (Maddrey and Weber, 1975).

Other metabolites derived from the diet which have been considered as causes of the cerebral syndrome include biogenic amines and indoles.

Studies by Livingstone et al. (1977), showing that in the hepatectomized rat, the blood brain barrier becomes permeable and compounds normally excluded, suggest that a similar situation may exist in hepatic failure. The various potential toxins elaborated by the bacteria in the intestine would then be particularly liable to reach target areas in the brain.

SELECTED REFERENCES

Arky, R.A., Veverbrants, E.A. and Abramson, E.A. 1968. Irreversible hypoglycemia; a complication of alcohol and insulin. J. Amer. Med. Assoc. 206: 575-578.

Baker, H., Luisada-Opper, A., Sorrell, M.F., Thomson, A.D. and Frank, O. 1973. Inhibition of nicotinic acid of hepatic steatosis and alcohol dehydrogenase in ethanol-treated rats. Exp. Molec. Pathol. 19: 106-112.

Balcerzak, S.P., Westerman, M.P. and Heinle, E.W. 1968. Mechanism of anemia in Zieve's syndrome. Amer. J. Med. Sci. 255: 277-287.

Baraona, E. and Lieber, C.S. 1969. Fatty liver, hyperlipemia and erythrocyte alterations produced by ethanol feeding in the rat. Amer. J. Clin. Nutr. 20: 356-357.

Becker, C.E., Roe, R.L. and Scott, R.A. 1974. *Alcohol as a Drug*. Baltimore: Williams and Wilkins Co. p. 26.

Benedetto, A.V., Kushner, J.P. and Taylor, J.S. 1978. Porphyria cutanea tarda in three generations of a single family. New Eng. J. Med. 298: 358-362.

Berggren, S.M. and Goldenberg, L. 1940. The absorption of ethyl alcohol from the gastrointestinal tract as a diffusion process. Acta Physiol. Scand. 1: 246-270.

Blass, J.P. and Dean, H.M. 1966. Relation of hyperlipemia to hemolytic anemia in an alcoholic patient. Amer. J. Med. 40: 283-289.

Bloom, E.R., Jr. 1976. The hepatic porphyrias. Pathogenesis, manifestations and management. Gastroenterology 71: 689-701.

Bogorad, L. 1963. Enzymatic mechanisms in porphyrin synthesis: possible enzymatic blocks in porphyrins. Ann. New York Acad. Sci. 104: 676-688.

Collier, H.B. 1952. Factors affecting the hemolytic action of "lysolecithin" upon rabbit erythrocytes. J. Gen. Physiol. 35: 617-628.

Cooper, R.A. and Shattil, S.J. 1971. Mechanisms of hemolysis - the minimal red cell defect. New Eng. J. Med. 285: 1514-1520.

Crouse, J.R., Gerson, C.D., DeCarli, L.M. and Leiber, C.S. 1968. Role of acetate in the reduction of plasma free fatty acids produced by ethanol in man. J. Lipid Res. 9: 509-512.

Dalmau-Ciria, M. 1962. Zieve's syndrome. Med. Clin. (Barc.) 39: 310-313.

De Matteis, P. 1967. Disturbances of liver porphyrin metabolism caused by drugs. Pharmacol. Rev. 19: 523-557.

Eales, L. 1963. Porphyria as seen in Capetown. A survey of 250 patients and some recent studies. S. Afr. J. Lab. Clin. Med. 9: 151-161.

Eales, L. 1971. Acute porphyria: The precipitating and aggravating factors. S. Afr. J. Lab. CLin. Med. 17: 120-125.

Eichner, E.R. 1973. The hematologic disorders of alcoholism. Amer. J. Med. 54: 621-630.

Eichner, E.R. and Hillman, R.S. 1971. The evolution of anemia in alcoholic patients. Amer. J. Med. 50: 218-232.

Eisner, M. and Berger, W. 1971. Biguanides and gastric emptying in man. Digestion IV: 309-313.

Elmslie, R.G., Davis, R.A., Magee, D.F. and White, T.T. 1965. Absorption of alcohol after gastrectomy. Surg. Gynecol. Abst. 119: 1256-1258.

Faloon, W.W. 1972. Hepatic mechanisms in pathophysiology. IN *Altered Regulatory Mechanisms in Disease*, Ed. Frohlich, E.D. Philadelphia: J.B. Lippincott Co. pp. 465-467.

Feuerlein, W. 1977. Neuropsychiatric disorders of alcoholism. Nutr. Metab. 21: 163-174.

Flink, E.B. 1971. Mineral metabolism, IN *The Biology of Alcoholism.* Vol. I, Biochemistry. Eds. Kissin, B. and Begleiter, H. New York: Plenum Press. pp. 377-395.

Flink, E.B., McCollister, R., Prasad, A.S., Melby, J.C. and Doe, P. 1957. Evidences for clinical magnesium deficiency. Ann. Intern. Med. 47: 956-968.

Flink, E.B., Shane, S.R., Jacobs, W.H. and Jovans, J.E. 1969. Some aspects of magnesium deficiency and chronic alcoholism, IN *Biochemical and Clinical Aspects of Alcohol Metabolism.* Springfield, IL: Charles C. Thomas Co. pp. 247-258.

Flink, E.B., Stutzman, F.L., Anderson, A.R., Konign, T. and Frazier, R. 1954. Magnesium deficiency after prolonged parenteral fluid administration and after chronic alcoholism complicated by delirium tremens. J. Lab. Clin. Med. 43: 169-183.

Forsander, O., Räihä, N. and Suomalainen, H. 1960. Oxydation des Äthylalkohols in Isolierter Leber und Isoliertem Hinterkörper der Ratte. Hoppe Seylers Z. Physiol. Chem. 318:1-5.

Franco, D., Deporte, A., Durandy, Y. and Bismuth, H. 1977. Upper gastrointestinal hemorrhage in hepatic cirrhosis: Causes and relation to hepatic failure and stress. Lancet 1: 218-220.

Frolich, E.D. 1972. Editor. Pathophysiology. *IN Altered Regulatory Mechanisms in Disease.* Philadelphia: J.B. Lippincott Co. p. 414.

Fukuda, R. 1964. A case of alcoholic fatty liver with Zieve's syndrome. J. Jap. Soc. Intern. Med. 52: 1495-1499.

Gibson, H.V. and Doisy, D.A. 1923. A note on the effect of some organic acids upon the uric acid excretion of man. J. Biol. Chem. 55: 605-610.

Gifford, H. and Turkel, H.W. 1956. Diffusion of alcohol through stomach wall after death. A cause of erroneous post mortem blood alcohol levels. J. Amer. Med. Assoc. 161: 866-868.

Goldberg, A. and Rimington, C. 1962. *Diseases of Porphyria Metabolism.* Springfield, IL.: Charles C. Thomas Co.

Goldfinger, S., Klinenberg, J.R. and Seegmiller, J.E. 1965. Renal retention of uric acid induced by infusion of beta-hydroxybutyrate and aceto acetate. New Eng. J. Med. 272: 351-355.

Golding, D.N. 1970. Alcohol-induced hypoglycaemia in childhood. Brit. Med. J. I: 278-280.

Haber, I. 1961. Zieve's syndrome: Report of a case. Acti. Gastro-interol. Belg. 24: 251-261.

Haberman, H.F., Rosenberg, F. and Mennan, I.A. 1975. Porphyria cutanea tarda: Comparison of cases precipitated by alcohol and estrogens. C.M.A.J. 4: 653-655.

Haggard, H.W. and Greenberg, L.A. 1934. Studies in the absorption, distribution, and elimination of ethyl alcohol. III. Rate of oxidation of alcohol in the body. J. Pharm. Exp. Therap. 52: 167-178.

Haggard, H.W. and Greenberg, L.A. 1940. Studies on the absorption, distribution, and elimination of alcohol. V. Influence of glycocol upon the absorption of alcohol. J. Pharmacol. 68: 482-493.

Haggard, H.W., Greenberg, L.A. and Cohen, L.H. 1938. Quantitative differences in the effects of alcoholic beverages. New Eng. J. Med. 219: 466-470.

Harger, R.N. and Hulpieu, H.R. 1935. Extent of absorption of alcohol at various intervals after oral administration. Proc. Soc. Exp. Biol. Med. 32: 1247-1249.

Hedding, R.C., Tothill, P., McLoughlin, G.P. and Shearman, D.J.C. 1974. Gastric emptying rate measurement in man: A method for simultaneous study of solid and liquid phases. Gut 15: 841.

Heggarty, H.J. 1970. Acute alcoholic hypoglycaemia in two 4-year-olds. Brit. Med. J. 1: 280.

Hillbroom, M.E. 1971. Regulation of hepatic elimination of ethanol *in vivo.* FEBS Lett. 17: 303-305.

Hopkins, A. 1966. The pattern of gastric emptying: A new view of old results. J. Physiol. 182: 114-149.

Hunt, J.N. 1960. The site receptors slowing gastric emptying in response to starch in test meals. J. Physiol. 154: 270-276.

Hunt, J.N. and MacDonald, K. 1954. The influence of volume of gastric emptying. J. Physiol. 126: 459-474.

Hunt, J.N. and Pathak, J.D. 1960. The osmotic effects of some simple molecules and ions on gastric emptying. J. Physiol. 154: 254-269.

Iseri, O.A., Gottlieb, L.S. and Lieber, C.S. 1964. The ultra-structure of fatty liver induced by prolonged ethanol ingestion. Fed. Proc. 23: 579.

Iseri, O.A., Lieber, C.S. and Gottlieb, L.S. 1966. The ultra-structure of fatty liver induced by prolonged ethanol ingestion. Amer. J. Pathol. 48: 535-555.

Isselbacher, K.J. 1977. Metabolic and hepatic effects of alcohol. New Eng. J. Med. 296: 612-616.

Isselbacher, K.J. and Greenberger, M.J. 1964. Metabolic effects of alcohol on the liver. New Eng. J. Med. 270: 351-410 and 402-410.

Jacob, H.S. and Amsden, T. 1971. Acute hemolytic anemia with rigid red cells in hypophosphatemia. New Eng. J. Med. 285: 1446-1450.

Jones, D.P. 1969. Effects of ethanol on lipid transport in man. IN *Biochemical and Clinical Aspects of Alcohol Metabolism*, Ed. Sardesai, V.M. Springfield, IL: Charles C. Thomas Co. pp. 86-94.

Kalant, H. 1971. Absorption, diffusion, distribution, and elimination of alcohol: Effects on biological membranes. IN *The Biology of Alcoholism*, Vol. 1, Biochemistry. Eds. Kissin, B. and Begleiter, H. New York: Plenum Press. pp. 1-62.

Karel, L. and Fleisher, J.H. 1948. Gastric absorption of ethyl alcohol in the rat. Amer. J. Physiol. 153: 268-276.

Kater, R.H., Carulli, N. and Iber, F.L. 1969. Differences in the rate of ethanol metabolism in recent drinking alcoholic and non-alcoholic subjects. Amer. J. Clin. Nutr. 22: 1608-1617.

Kessel, L. 1962. Acute transient hyperlipemia due to hemopoietal pancreatic damage in chronic alcoholics (Zieve's syndrome). Amer. J. Med. 32: 747-757.

Knudson, K.B., Sparberg, M. and Lecocq, F. 1967. Porphyria precipitated by fasting. New Eng. J. Med. 277: 350-351.

Krebs, H.A. 1968. The effect of ethanol on the metabolic activities of the liver. Adv. Enzyme Regula. 6: 467-480.

Krebs, H.A. 1974. The metabolism of ethanol. IN *Topics in Gastroenterology*. Eds. Truelove, S.C. and Trowell, J. Oxford and London: Blackwell Scientific Publishers.

Larsen, J.A. Elimination of ethanol as a measure of the hepatic blood flow in the cat. II. The significance of the extra hepatic elimination of ethanol. Acta Physiol. Scand. 57: 209-223.

Lecocq, F.R. and McPhaul, J.J. Jr. 1965. The effects of starvation, high fat diets and ketone infusions on uric acid balance. Metabolism 14: 186-197.

Leevy, C.M., Cardi, L., Frank, O., Gellene, R. and Baker, H. 1965. Incidence in significant hypovitaminemia in a randomly selected municipal hospital for population. Amer. J. Clin. Nutr. 17: 259-271.

Leevey, C.M., Tamburro, C., Kirklan, M. and Cabasag, C. 1969. Biochemical alterations in delirium tremens. IN *Biochemical and Clinical Aspects of Alcohol Metabolism*, Ed. Sardesai, V.M. Springfield, IL: Charles C. Thomas Publ. Co. 1969. 241-246.

Levine, R.R. 1973. *Pharmacology - Drug Actions and Reactions*. Boston: Little, Brown and Co. p. 80.

Levy, G. and Jusko, W.J. 1965. Effect of viscosity on drug absorption. J. Pharm. Sci. 54: 219-225.

Lieber, C.S. 1975. Interference of ethanol in hepatic cellular metabolism. Ann. New York Acad. Sci. 25: 24-50.

Lieber, C.S. and DeCarli, L.M. 1968. Ethanol oxidation by hepatic microsomes: Adaptive increase after ethanol feeding. Science 162: 917-918.

Lieber, C.S. and DeCarli, L.M. 1970. Hepatic microsomal ethanol-oxidizing system: In vitro characteristics and adaptive properties in vivo. J. Biol. Chem. 245: 2505-2512.

Lieber, C.S., Jones, D.P., DeCarli, L.M. 1965. Effects of prolonged ethanol intake: Production of fatty liver despite adequate diets. J. Clin. Invest. 44: 1009-1021.

Lieber, C.S., Jones, D.P. Losowsky, M.S. and Davidson, C.S. 1962. Interrelation of uric acid in ethanol metabolism in man. J. Clin. Invest. 41: 1863-1870.

Lieber C.S., Leevy, C.M., Stein, S.W., George, W.S., Cherrick, G.R., Abelman, W.H. and Davidson, D.S. 1962b. Effect of ethanol on plasma free fatty acids in man. J. Lab. Clin. Med. 59: 826-832.

Lieber, C.S. and Rubin, E. 1968. Alcoholic fatty liver in man on a high protein and low fat diet. Amer. J. Med. 44: 200-206.

Lieber, C.S., Teschke, R., Hasumura, Y. and DeCarli, L.M. 1975. Differences in hepatic and metabolic changes after acute and chronic alcohol consumption. Fed. Proc. 34: 2060-2074.

Livingstone, A.S., Potvin, M., Goresky, C.A., Finlayson, M.H. and Hinchey, E.J. 1977. Changes in the blood-brain barrier in hepatic coma after hepatectomy in the rat. Gastroenterology 73: 697-704.

Lunduist, F. and Wolthers, H. 1958. The kinetics of alcohol elimination in man. Acta Pharm. Tox., KBH 14: 265-289.

Lundsgaard, E. 1938. Alcohol oxidation as a function of the liver. C.R. Lab. Carlsberg Ser. Chem. 22: 333-337.

Lundvall, O., Weinfield, A. and Lundin, P. 1970. Iron storage in porphyria cutanea tarda. Acta Med. Scand. 188: 37-53.

Lynn, Y-J., Weidler, D.J., Garg, D.C. and Wagner, J.G. 1976. Effects of solid food on blood levels of alcohol in man. Res. Commun. Chem. Pathol. Pharmacol. 13: 713-722.

MacLachlan, M.J. and Rodnan, P. 1967. Effects of food, fast and alcohol on serum uric acid and acute attacks of gout. Amer. J. Med. 42: 38-57.

Maddrey, W.C. and Weber, F.L. 1975. Chronic hepatic encephalopathy. Med. Clin. N. America 59: 937-944.

Madison, L.L. IN Advances in Metabolic Disorders, Vol. III. Eds. Levin, R. and Luft, R. London: Academic Press, p. 85.

Mellanby, E. 1919. Alcohol: Its absorption into and disappearance from the blood under different conditions. MRC Publ. Special Report Series 31, London: His Majesty's Stationery Office.

Mellanby, E. 1920. Alcohol and alcoholic intoxication. Brit. J. Inebr. 17: 157-178.

Mello, N.K. 1972. Behavioral studies of alcoholism. IN *The Biology of Alcoholism*. Vol. II: Physiology and Behavior. Eds. Kissin, B. and Begleiter, H. New York and London: Plenum Press. 219-291.

Mendelson, J.H. 1964. Experimentally induced chronic intoxication and withdrawal in alcoholics. Quart. J. Stud. Alc., Suppl. No. 2. 1-129.

Miles, W.R. 1922. The comparative concentrations of alcohol in human blood and urine at intervals after digestion. J. Pharmacol. Exper. Therap. 20: 265-319.

Miller, D.S. and Sterling, J.L. 1966. The effect of a meal on the rate of ethanol metabolism in man. Proc. Nutr. Soc. 25: X1.

Miller, D.S., Sterling, J.L. and Yudkin, J. 1966. Effect of ingestion of milk on concentrations of blood alcohol. Nature 212: 1051.

Myerson, R.M. 1973. Metabolic aspects of alcohol and their biological significance. Med. Clin. N. America 57: 925-940.

Orme-Johnson, W.H., and Ziegler, D.M. 1965. Alcohol mixed function oxidase activity of mammalian liver microsomes. Biochem. Biophys. Res. Comm. 21: 78-82.

Oshino, N., Oshino, R. and Chance, B. 1973. The characteristics of the "peroxidatic" reaction of catalase in ethanol oxidation. Biochem. J. 131: 555-563.

Payne, J.P., Hill, D.W. and King, N.W. 1966. Observations on the distribution of alcohol in blood, breath and urine. Brit. Med. J. I: 196-202.

Petite, J.P 1964. Zieve's syndrome. Presse Med. 72: 1501-1507.

Plueckhahn, V.D. and Ballard, B. 1967. Diffusion of stomach alcohol and heart blood alcohol concentration at autopsy. J. Forensic Sci. 12: 463-470.

Popper, H. 1976. Cirrhosis, Alcohol and the Liver. Proc. Canadian Hepatic Foundation 3rd Internat. Symp., Toronto, May 14-15. 1976. Ed. Fisher, M.M. and Rankin, J.G. New York: Plenum Press.

Powell, L.W., Roeser, H.P. and Haliday, J.W. 1972. Transient intravascular hemolysis associated with alcoholic liver disease and hyperlipidaemia. Aust. N.Z. J. Med. 1: 39-43.

Robinson, N. 1961. Lysolecithin. J. Pharm. Pharmacol. 13: 321-354.

Rose, J.A., Helman, E.S. and Tschudy, D.P. 1961. Effect of diet on induction of experimental porphyria. Metabolism 10: 514-521.

Rubin, E., Bacchin, P., Gang, H., and Lieber, C.S. 1970. Induction and inhibition of hepatic microsomal mitochrondrial enzymes by ethanol. Lab. Invest. 22: 569-580.

Rubin, E. and Lieber, C.S. 1967. Early fine structural changes in the human liver induced by alcohol. Gastroenterology 52: 1-13.

Rubin, E. and Lieber, C.S. 1968. Alcohol-induced hepatic injury in non-alcoholic volunteers. New Eng. J. Med. 278: 869-876.

Rubin, E. and Lieber, C.S. 1974. Fatty liver, alcoholic hepatitis and cirrhosis produced by alcohol in primates. New Eng. J. Med. 290: 128-135.

Salvesen, H. and Kolberg, A. 1958. Alcohol absorption in idiopathic steator-rhea. Acta Med. Scand. 161: 135-142.

Sarles, H. 1977. Alcohol in the pancreas. Nutr. Metab. 21: 175-186.

Schmidt, M. 1934. Alcohol studies. II. Concentration of alcohol in the blood. J. Indust. Hyg. 16: 355-365.

Scholz, R. and Nohl, H. 1976. Mechanism of the stimulatory effect of fructose on ethanol oxidation in perfused rat liver. Europ. J. Biochem. 63: 449-458.

Scott, J.T., McCallum, F.M. and Holloway, V.P. 1964. Starvation, ketosis and uric acid excretion. Clin. Sci. 27: 209-221.

Sedman, A.J., Wilkinson, P.K., Sakmar, E., Weidler, D. and Wagner, J.G. 1976. Food effects on absorption and metabolism of alcohol. Quart. J. Stud. Alc. 37: 1197-1214.

Seegmiller, J.E. 1974. Diseases of pyrroline and pyrimidine metabolism. IN *Duncan's Diseases of Metabolism*, 7th ed. Eds. Bondy, P.K. and Rosenberg, L.E. Philadelphia: W.B. Saunders Co. p.679.

Sellers, E.M. and Kalant, H. 1976. Alcohol intoxication and withdrawal. New Eng. J. Med. 294: 757-762.

Serianni, E., Cannizzaro, M., and Mariani, A. 1953. Blood alcohol concentrations resulting from wine drinking timed according to the dietary habits of Italians. Quart. J. Stud. Alc. 14: 165-173.

Sherlock, S. 1963. *Diseases of the Liver and Biliary System*, 3rd ed. Philadelphia: F.A. Davis Co. pp. 100-101.

Smith, J.A., Lonergan, E.T. and Sterling, K. 1964. Spur cell anemia: Hemolytic anemia with red cells resembling acanthocytes in alcoholic cirrhosis. New Eng. J. Med. 271: 396-401.

Stege, T.E., Hanby, J.D. and DiLuzio, N.R. 1976. Acetaldehyde-induced hepatic lipid peroxidation. IN *Currents in Alcoholism, Biological, Biochemical and Clinical Studies.* Vol. 1, Ed. Seixas, F.A. New York: Grune and Stratton. pp. 139-159.

Strom, J. 1963. Zieve's syndrome. Report of a case. Acta Med. Scand. 174: 219-222.

Thompson, J.N. 1965. Some aspects of the metabolism and biochemistry of vitamin A. Proc. Nutr. Soc. 24: 160-166.

Thurman, R.G. 1973. Quantitative assessment of the role of catalase-H_2O_2 in ethanol utilization by perfused rat liver. Fed. Proc. 32: 1429.

Timme, A.H. 1971. The ultrastructure of the liver in human symptomatic porphyria: A preliminary communication. S. Afr. J. Lab. Clin. Med. 17: 58-72. (Special Issue).

Timme, A.H., Dowdle, E.B. and Eales, L. 1974. Symptomatic porphyria. I. The pathology of the liver in human symptomatic porphyria. S. Afr. Med. J. 48: 1803-1807.

Tschudy, D.P. 1975. Acute intermittent porphyria: Clinical and selected research aspects. Ann. Intern. Med. 83: 851-864.

Turnbull, A. 1971. On metabolism in the porphyrias. Brit. J. Dermat. 84: 380-383.

Ugarte, G., Iturriaga, H. and Pereda, T. 1977. Possible relationship between the rate of ethanol metabolism and the severity of hepatic damage in chronic alcoholics. Dig. Dis. 22: 406-410.

Ugarte, G., Pereda, T., Pino, M.E. and Iturriaga, H. 1972. Influence of alcohol intake, length of abstinence and meprobamate on the rate of ethanol metabolism in men. Quart. J. Stud. Alc. 33: 698-705.

Ulys, C.J. and Eales, L. 1963. The histopathology of the liver in acquired (symptomatic) porphyria. S. Afr. J. Lab. Clin. Med. 9: 190-197.

Videla, L. and Israel, V. 1970. Factors that modify the metabolism of ethanol in the rat liver and adaptive changes produced by its chronic administration. Biochem. J. 118: 275-281.

Voltz, W., Baudrexel, A. and Dietrich, W. 1912. Über die vom tierischen organismus unter verschiedenen bedingungen ausgeschiedenen alkohol mengen. III. Einfluss des füllungszustandes des magen-darm-kanals auf die alkoholausschiedung in harn und atmung. Arch. Ges. Physiol. 145: 210-228.

von Wartburg, J.P. 1971. The metabolism of alcohol in normals and alcoholics: Enzymes. IN The Biology of Alcoholism, Vol.1 Biochemistry. Eds. Kissin, B. and Begleiter, H. New York: Plenum Press. pp. 63-102.

von Wartburg, J.P. 1977. Metabolic consequences of alcohol consumption. Nutr. Metab. 21: 153-162.

Waldo, E.D. and Tobias, H. 1973. Needle-like cytoplasmic inclusions in the liver in porphyria cutanea tarda. Arch. Pathol. 96: 368-371.

Walters, P.R. and Owen, P. 1963. Pancreatic enzymes and intra-vascular hemolysis. Blood 22: 812-813.

Welland, F.H., Hellman, E.S., Gaddis, E.M., Collins, A., Hunter, G.W. Jr., and Tschudy, D.P. 1964. Factors affecting excretion of porphyrin precursors by patients with acute intermittent porphyria. I. Effect of diet. Metabolism 13: 232-250.

Welling, P.G. 1977. Influence of food and drugs on gastrointestinal drug absorption: A review. J. Pharmacokinet. Biopharmacent. V: 291-334.

Westerman, M.P., Balcerzak, S.P. and Heinle, E.W. 1968. Red cell lipids in Zieve's syndrome: Their relation to hemolysis and to red cell osmotic fragility. J. Lab. Clin. Med. 72: 663-670.

Whitcomb, H.C. and Job, H.J. 1960. Zieve's syndrome: A case report. Rocky Mountain M.J. 57: 49-52.

Widmarck, E.M.P. 1933. Über die einwirkung von aminosäuren auf den alkoholgehalt des blutes. Biochem. Z. 265: 237-240.

Widmarck, E.M.P. 1933b. Der einflüss der nahrungesbestandteile auf den alkoholgehalt des blutes. Biochem. Z. 267: 135-142.

Widmarck, E.M.P. 1935. Hormonal einflüsse auf den alkoholumsatz. Biochem. Z. 282: 79-84.

Wolfe, S.M. and Victor, M. 1969. The relationship of hypomagnesemia and alcolysis to alcohol withdrawal symptoms. Ann. New York Acad. Sci. 162: 973-984.

Zieve, L. 1958. Jaundice, hyperlipemia and hemolytic anemia: A hither-to-for unrecognized syndrome associated with alcoholic fatty liver and cirrhosis. Ann. Int. Med. 48: 471-496.

Zieve, L. and Hill, E. 1959. Hemolytic anemia in cirrhosis. South. Med. J. 52: 903-911.

Zieve, L. and Hill, E. 1961. Two varieties of hemolytic anemia in cirrhosis. South. Med. J. 54: 1347-1352.

4

Eating Behavior of Social Drinkers and Indigent Alcoholics

Among drinkers as well as non-drinkers, determinants of food choice and eating times can be considered as either of sociocultural or environmental origin. While the substance and manner in which anyone eats is influenced by cultural, social, personal, and situational factors, and whereas such groups of factors collectively determine what and when a person eats, within this classification drinkers are more influenced by situational variation than non-drinkers.

Major cultural factors which determine eating practices are the sociocultural group of origin, which includes ethnicity, country of origin, religious beliefs, familiar foods, food taboos, foods believed to alter destiny or health, as well as drinking and eating practices followed by the particular culture.

Social factors which influence eating practices include the habits of the parents, the influence of the family, upward social mobility or downward social trends, the emotional association of foods, and foods which are considered by the group to which the individual belongs, as being appropriate to particular meals and occasions. Since drinking occasions may be one and the same with eating occasions, eating behaviors of the drinkers will be influenced by foods commonly available at luncheons, dinners, cocktail parties, group meetings, and a variety of festive holidays.

Personal factors which influence eating practices include early association, taste satisfaction, and sensory pleasure derived from foods. It is to be noted that in alcoholics, early satiety, taste impairment and aversive responses to food may limit or alter the range or amount of foods consumed. Desire to eat, and to enjoy food, may be tempered by the responses that food evokes; more particularly, when alcohol-related diseases are present, especially those pertaining to the gastrointestinal tract.

Very many situational factors condition what a social drinker or alcoholic eats on a day-to-day or week-to-week basis. These include his/her mental state, whether there is a sense of happiness or euphoria, whether the person is anxious or depressed, as well as anger, placidity and agitation. Whereas it is well established that psychotic depression is usually followed by or associated with loss of appetite, neurotic depression is frequently associated with an excessive intake of food, or an actual food addiction. Physical health has a profound influence on eating behavior. In the alcoholic, morning nausea (or nausea on waking) cannot only be considered in terms of the after-effects of intoxication, but also as a common sign of impending or existing liver disease including hepatitis and cirrhosis. Statements such as "I used to eat breakfast regularly, but now I don't feel like it." or "I can't stomach the sight of food in the morning." are particularly characteristic of those alcoholics who have recently gotten out of control; those who begin to drink in the early hours of the morning because of early withdrawal symptoms or insomnia, and those with impaired liver function. Binge drinkers may report inability to eat breakfast on the day after a spree, or a need to eat later in the morning may be rationalized. Alcoholics in a hypomanic phase of a manic-depressive illness may arise early in the morning and go on long walks, roaming city streets in search of company, food, and drink. Clearly, circumstances do affect such behaviors for, whereas the city dweller may be able to satisfy his/her early morning food and drink requirements in or around a marketplace, such opportunities may not present themselves to someone living in a rural area. It is noticeable that the mental "high" may override coexistent effects of alcohol-related diseases which might otherwise suppress appetite for food in the early morning.

Income or food budget is an important determinant. Among low income individuals the food budget may be severely reduced when the habit of alcohol abuse is also supported. It has come to the author's attention that in recent times, alcoholics on public assistance may sell Food Stamps in order to get money to purchase liquor. As the food budget is reduced, the ability to obtain variety in the diet is also lost and the more expensive foods, including fresh meats, fish, cheese, fruits and many vegetables, become luxury items. As the diet becomes less diversified, because of reduced intake of these foods, so the likelihood of nutrient imbalances increases and the opportunities for the individual to obtain an adequate nutrient intake decline. In the binge-drinking alcoholic, the food budget may be sufficient except at times when liquor purchases or purchases of other alcoholic beverages rise above available income.

The alcoholic's economic status may fluctuate markedly from time to time, with change in work status, marital status, and eligibility for welfare assistance. If the job is lost through alcohol abuse or if the marital or sex partner who offers financial support leaves, or if it is considered that the alcoholic is abusing the welfare system, then income may be more and more constrained and the ability to purchase food of adequate quality and quantity is diminished. At the same time, the alcoholic may move into a one-room apartment, not offering cooking facilities, or into a hotel or rooming house which does not supply meals. Under any of these unsatisfactory living conditions, food choices are not only limited by the amount of money available, but also by constraints related to food purchase, storage, and preparation. We are accustomed to the indigent or low income alcoholic whose food sources and eating places are limited to vending machines, snack bars, fast food counters, and diners. Dietary deficiencies and excesses are then related to the foods available, and particularly the food that can be bought most cheaply. Skid row alcoholics are, however, likely to avail themselves of community meals offered either at no cost or at nominal price, as well as foods distributed by churches and other philanthropic institutions. While these accessory food sources offer supplementary nourishment of variable quality, it can be generalized that their basic foods are more likely to be canned soups, canned meats, and bread or crackers, rather than fresh foods such as vegetables or fruits.

Alcoholics' occupations may determine eating times and actual foods consumed. The alcoholic business person is likely to be a victim of circumstance when he/she succumbs to temptations of food excesses. Business lunches, cocktail parties, dinners and other social occasions at which liquor is served, offer the alcoholic opportunities to readily exceed an intake above energy requirements, and also to consume excess salt, fat, and high cholesterol foods. The alcoholic working at a fast-food counter or other food service establishment is likely to eat those foods which are available at little or no cost to employees at times when eating is permitted. Alcoholic bartenders or others who successfully maintain occupational contact with alcohol, are likely to eat most of what is available at work, including crackers, potato chips and other snack foods.

It is not only occupational contact with alcohol that determines eating practices, but also occupational knowledge of nutrition may influence food intake. Thus, alcohol-addicted individuals in health professions, who have a basic knowledge of nutrition, may be regularly inclined to eat a diet endowed in their minds with health-giving properties. Attempts may be made to offset the toxic effects of ethanol by consumption of foods rich in vitamins or other nutrients. On the other hand, alcoholic physicians, health scientists and scientific writers may follow a particular dietary regimen as prophylaxis against diet-related disease such as atherosclerosis or hypertension.

Eating and drinking times in the alcoholic, as in the non-alcoholic, are markedly influenced by the work timetable. Actors, private duty nurses, night porters and nightwatchmen may eat almost entirely after dark, consuming their alcoholic beverages of choice over this same time period. The foods consumed by people in these occupations are determined by availability, convenience in preparation, and the presence or absence of cooking facilities.

Health variables certainly affect eating habits of alcoholics. Thus, morning nausea with or without anorexia may determine whether or not a breakfast is eaten. Aversive responses to particular foods will also condition their elimination from the diet. For example, if an alcoholic has a lactose intolerance, he/she may stop drinking milk. Similarly, alcohol-related taste perversions may alter food choice. Alcoholics with secondary diseases may be on restricted diets, either because these are self-imposed, or advised by a physician. Fatty foods may be restricted in alcoholics with chronic pancreatitis. The alcoholic with a peptic ulcer may limit intake of coffee, or those with diarrhea and other bowel symptoms may be placed on a low residue diet. We are impressed that alcoholics vary in their compliance with dietary regimes, but may follow the diet to a letter with the exception that they continue to consume alcoholic beverages to excess.

COMPLEX CULTURAL FACTORS AFFECTING EATING AND DRINKING PRACTICES

It is known that in certain countries and cultures, specific alcoholic beverages, such as wine or beer, may be considered as food rather than as intoxicants. Studies by Luzzatto-Fegiz and Lolli (1957) of the attitudes of Italians toward the drinking of milk and wine illustrate such viewpoints. Their study population were living in northern, central and southern Italy as well as on the Italian islands. While 9% of the respondents were described as being wealthy, 43% were middle-class and 48% were persons of low income. Findings of this study were that the majority of the Italians in the sample were not convinced that milk was an essential or health-giving food for adults, but that it was considered normal for adults to drink wine with meals. In fact, large amounts of wine were consumed with main meals and also between meals. The drinking of milk was largely confined to breakfast, and at that time it was usually taken with coffee. Asked how much wine should be taken by different people engaged in occupations requiring large or small amounts of physical activity, the concensus was that for individuals engaged in heavy manual labor, it was believed that an average of 1.4 liters of wine could safely be consumed daily and that for those engaged in doing light work, only eight-tenths of a liter of wine was considered to be appropriate. Authors conclude from these responses that Italians within this group believe that wine is an energy-yielding food and as such, would be required more by those doing heavy manual work. It was further found that the nourishing qualities of wine were more accepted by men than by women, and more by older people than by young respondents.

Additional observations of these authors were that the largest consumption of wine with main meals (that is, lunch and dinner), were observed among farmers and farm laborers, and the smallest among white-collar workers and housewives. Reasons given for not drinking milk with lunch or dinner were "I don't like it"; "I don't like it while I eat"; "I'm not in the habit of using milk"; or "I prefer wine." Among respondents, 61% believed that wine is nourishing, 79% believed that wine gives strength, and 15% believed that wine is more nourishing than milk. In addition, 26% believed that good wine is harmless, even if consumed in considerable amounts. Among 1,453 persons who were involved in this investigation, only one thought that the drinking of wine could lead to alcoholism.

Beginning in 1952, Lolli et al. studied and compared the eating and drinking practices of Italians living in Italy and Italian-Americans. In both groups history showed that wine had been consumed with meals since childhood. The Italian group drank wine regularly with meals, the Italian-Americans tended to drink wine less regularly, or on an intermittent basis, and also to consume other alcoholic beverages. Drinking between meals was more common in the Italian-Americans than in the Italians. Attitudes toward wine were sought from the parents of respondents in the sample, who consisted of persons living either in Rome or in New Haven, Connecticut. Italian-born parents who were living in Italy did not question the wisdom of drinking wine. They considered wine as a food, and according to the authors, "probably a basic element of the diet, like bread or vegetables." First generation Italian parents who had immigrated to the U.S. were quite positive in their attitudes toward the value of wine. It was surmised that they desired to preserve customs, traditional of the Italian culture. Several of the respondents had recollections of drunkenness in early youth. Of the 50 Italian subjects, only seven had had more than six episodes of drunkenness in their lifetimes, and of these, only one was considered to be an alcoholic. Among the 44 Italian-American subjects, multiple episodes of excessive drinking that were reported were infrequent in most subjects, and in this group there was only one addictive drinker. However, the definition of addiction by these authors is perhaps somewhat unusual, in that they state "The quality which characterizes the addictive drinker is his disposition to react to the effects of alcohol in such a way that some of his anomalous and pressing needs are satisfied, albeit, briefly and inadequately. The personality of the addictive drinker is so oriented that he seeks and is able to experience by means of alcohol a unique pleasure, wherein physiological satisfactions are inexplicably blended with psychological ones, the latter being characterized by the possibility at a given blood alcohol concentration, of simultaneously expressing contradictory emotions... Addiction becomes patent only when the individual discovers that alcohol and alcohol alone satisfies that longing for a blended pleasure of body and mind which is typical of his deviant personality."

Considerable variability was found in the percent of total calories from all alcoholic beverages that were consumed, such that both in the Italians and in the Italian-Americans, alcohol contribution to total calories only exceeded 15% in three Italians (two men, one woman) and in the Italian-Americans, two subjects (one man, one woman). In most subjects the percentage caloric intake from alcohol was estimated to be less than 5%.

In a further study by Lolli et al. (1953), 300 subjects were interrogated including 89 Italian men, 58 Italian women, 73 Italian-American men and 80 Italian-American women. Several differences were observed between the drinking and eating habits of Italians and Italian-Americans. Italians drank wine more frequently and consistently than the Italian-Americans in the week in which food and alcohol intakes were recorded, and the amounts of wine taken contributed a significant· portion of the total energy intake. Few of the Italians drank beer during the week of observation, though Italian-Americans consumed beer in larger amounts. Liquor was not consumed in appreciable amounts by the Italians, but was taken by a number of the Italian-American subjects. Drinking exclusively with meals was the norm among the Italians, but the Italian-Americans showed diversified drinking patterns with various combinations of drinking and eating existing among this group, suggesting partial acclimatization to the

American culture. In this study, drinking histories suggested that the number of men and women who had never been intoxicated was higher among Italians than among the Italian-Americans.

These studies of Italians and Italian-Americans suggest that social acceptance of wine drinking and the drinking of wine at meal-times is perhaps a deterrent to alcohol addiction. However, it is well known that in France, where wine is also drunk with meals, alcoholism is a major public health problem. Apparent differences in the incidences of alcoholism in wine drinking countries stem from different definitions of alcohol abuse, or greater or earlier recognition of the early signs of alcoholism in one country as compared with another. Delore (1953), who emphasized alcoholism as a "major scourge in France," intimated that if you could promote the drinking of fruit juice in France, alcohol consumption could decline.

Whereas acceptance of wine drinking as a normal accompaniment of meals was previously considered as a possible deterrent to alcoholism, reality does not support this thesis. Solms (1976) documents that in wine drinking countries, including France, Portugal, Italy and Spain, the mortality from cirrhosis of the liver is greater than in non-wine drinking countries.

Pequignot (1963), Pequignot and Cyrulnik (1970), and Lelbach (1974) have demonstrated that there is a highly significant correlation between alcohol dosage, time (that is, over-consumption over a long period), and the toxic effects of alcohol. We must presume that, whether or not wine drinking is commonplace and an accompaniment of eating, it can no longer be accepted that the consumption of wine with full meals prevents alcoholic diseases or mortality. In France, where the mortality from cirrhosis is higher than in other European countries (Solms, 1976), ingestion of liquor between meals and brandies or other liquors after meals does contribute to total alcohol intake.

EATING HABITS OF BINGE DRINKERS

The most unsatisfactory aspect of the diets and eating habits of alcoholics has, in the past, been that there has not been an appropriate control group. We have recently had the opportunity to study the eating habits of a group of men and women on public assistance in Upstate New York (Roe, 1978). The total sample claimed medical problems as reasons why they could not work, or enter federal job training programs. Prominent medical problems identified in the group included neurosis, sick role behavior, back problems, obesity and its complications, late effects of injury or surgery, visual and hearing impairments, chronic cardiovascular and respiratory disease, and alcoholism or other substance abuse. Alcoholics were defined by drinking history, history of hospitalizations for detoxication, or alcohol-related diseases, and by mean corpuscular volume (greater than 93 cuμ) in the absence of macrocytic anemia. Supportive evidence was obtained from the diagnosis of alcohol-related diseases and laboratory findings indicative of alcoholic hepatitis or cirrhosis. Positive correlations were obtained between a history of alcohol abuse and elevation in mean corpuscular volume, and between alcohol abuse and elevated serum transaminase levels (SGOT and SGPT). Most of the alcoholics were "weekly heavy drinkers," according to the Knupfer classification (1966). Drinking was for the relief of tension, or for purposes of intoxication rather than for the social effect. Drinkers reported alcohol abuse one or more times per week, at which time they might consume a single beverage or several different types of alcoholic beverages including gin, whiskey, vodka, mixed drinks including sweet mixed drinks, as well as beer. Wine drinking was uncommon. Missed meals and irregular and low intake of vegetables were common findings in the total group, and did not distinguish alcoholics from non-alcoholics. Irregularity of missed meals during the week was significantly more common in the alcoholic subgroup who were also less likely to prepare or buy a lunch. Alcoholics also consumed raw vegetables less frequently than non-alcoholics, and candy less frequently than non-alcoholics. The possibility that lower consumption of candy by the alcoholics could be related to smoking was examined, but it was found that even controlling for smoking, alcoholics ate candy less frequently than the non-alcoholics in the group. Answers to the structured questionnaire did not allow us to discover whether dinners were missed by alcoholics at times of episodic drinking (Fig. 4.1).

In this study, three-day diet diaries were not satisfactory as a means of discovering patterns of eating and drinking in the heavy weekly drinkers. However, in studying alcoholics with cirrhosis of the liver, Olsen (1950) obtained a stereotyped answer to questions about effects of drinking on food consumption such that responses were uniformly "I eat poorly when drinking." Among our patients this was only true in those on prolonged alcoholic sprees, or in the few who were heavy daily drinkers. We suspect, but have not yet proven, that the pattern among the alcoholics was one of downward social mobility, whereas the non-alcoholic group came from a background of chronic poverty and unemployment. In support of this hypothesis was the finding that the employment histories of the alcoholics were better than those of the non-alcoholics with respect to job tenure.

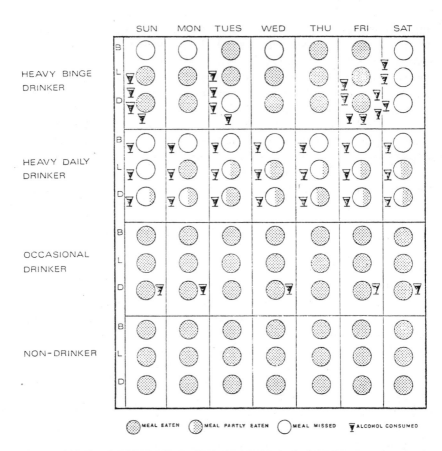

FIG. 4.1. SCHEMATIC REPRESENTATION OF RELATIONSHIPS BETWEEN DRINKING
AND MEAL CONSUMPTION IN HEAVY BINGE DRINKERS, HEAVY DAILY DRINKERS,
AND OCCASIONAL DRINKERS.

Irregular food habits as well as the consumption of diets of low
vitamin content have been stressed in the literature as commonplace
among chronic alcoholics (Neville *et al.*, 1968). Caution must be exercised in accepting this stereotype, though it may indeed be true of the
skid row alcoholic who is also a vagrant (Ashley *et al.*, 1976).

In 1953, Figueroa *et al.* made a dietary assessment and examined the
nutritional status of 451 men admitted to the House of Correction of
the City of Chicago. The actual survey was conducted between June,
1948 and July, 1949. In addition to the target group, nearly 16,000
inmates of this institution were screened for evidence of classical
nutritional deficiency syndromes. Among the 451 men who had been
newly admitted to the institution, 23% were markedly underweight.

Among these men, the investigators only found two with pellagra, one with possible beriberi, three with riboflavin deficiency, one with Wernicke's syndrome, and seven with other possible nutritional polyneuropathies. No overt cases of scurvy or vitamin A deficiency were detected. In the total group screened, evidence of florid vitamin deficiency was low. The authors, who were expecting to find a higher incidence of specific nutritional deficiencies among their target population, explained the relative lack of such findings as being due to the consumption of enriched bread and cereals by the alcoholics in the institutions. A comment is made that "Our 'average' alcoholic lives on coffee, donuts, bread, thick soups, spaghetti, stews, and hash. Many of them eat at least eight slices of bread a day. This would supply them with 5.3 mg of niacin, 0.7 mg of thiamin, and 0.5 mg of riboflavin." It is intimated that the intake of the fortified bread by the alcoholics, as well as other quantities of B vitamins obtained from the diet, would be adequate to prevent "florid nutritional deficiency disease." Findings are compared with earlier studies, before the enrichment of bread, indicating a high incidence of pellagra and other B vitamin deficiencies among alcoholics (Klauder and Winkelman, 1928; Spies and DeWolf, 1933; Texon, 1948).

Whereas it was concluded by Figueroa *et al.* (1953) that lack of florid avitaminoses among alcoholics was mainly due to their consumption of enriched bread, other factors may have contributed to the findings, including changes in economic status which may have occurred since the prewar studies were conducted. In addition, it should be pointed out that criteria for the diagnosis of vitamin deficiency among the alcoholics in the Chicago House of Correction may have failed to identify malnutrition when not accompanied by classical signs such as dermatoses.

Influence of Nutrient Intake on Alcohol Intake

More than 25 years ago, Williams elaborated the theory that alcoholism is a "genetotrophic disease," and that it arises in certain individuals who do not consume sufficient nutrients to meet their needs. This theory was based on observations of rats in which it was claimed that with a heterogeneous rat population, all animals on a marginal diet will consume ethanol, but as the diet approximates to the nutritional requirements of the animals within the population, so the alcohol appetite diminishes (Williams, 1953; Williams *et al.*, 1950).

Register *et al.* (1972) designed a study to determine whether administration of a "teen-age type diet," marginal in nutrients, to rats would elicit drinking behavior with respect to alcohol. Observations in this experiment suggested that animals fed diets that were deficient in vitamins had increased intakes of alcohol which, according to the authors, could be reversed by "adding the missing nutrient to the diet." While the present author does not support the hypothesis that alcohol craving is diet-dependent in the first place, alcohol addiction and food addiction may be related. Further, alcoholics faced with the choice of satisfying their appetite with alcoholic beverages or monotonous, ill-prepared food, may choose the former, whereas if they are offered well prepared and attractive meals, they may be induced to lower their alcohol consumption.

CIGARETTE SMOKING AND VITAMINS

The eating habits of alcoholics may be markedly influenced by their other habitual behaviors. In our own studies, and in those of several other investigators, alcohol abuse has been associated with smoking, both qualitatively and quantitatively (Health, 1958; Matarazzo and Saslow, 1960; Higgins et al., 1967). Alcohol consumption has also been correlated with coffee consumption (Friedman et al., 1974). There is strong reason to suspect, though presently it is unproven, that the eating habits of many alcoholics may be influenced by their concomitant smoking and heavy coffee consumption. As mentioned previously, we have found that alcoholics consume less sugar than nonalcoholics, and this may be explained on the basis of preference for cigarettes and/or coffee in place of desserts and candy.

Certain investigators, such as Neville et al. (1968), have noted that specific groups of alcoholics are in the habit of taking vitamin supplements on a regular basis. Vitamin supplements may be taken in excess of recommended dosages. No doubt many alcoholics believe that they will avoid the adverse effects of ethanol by partaking of these added nutrients. Indeed, such beliefs are fostered by purveyors of patent medicines containing vitamins and minerals who benefit most from this idea.

REFERENCES

Ashley, M.J., Olin, J.S., Harding le Riche, W., Kornaczewski, A., Schmidt, W., and Rankin, J.G. 1976. Skid row alcoholism: A distinct sociomedical entity. Arch. Int. Med. 136: 272-278.

Delore, P. 1953. Propo sur l'alcoolisme. Pr. Méd. 61: 537-538.

Figueroa, W. G., Sargent, F., Imperiale, L., Morey, G.R., Paynter, C.R. and Vorhaus, L.J. 1953. Lack of avitaminosis among alcoholics. J. Clin. Nutr. 1: 179-199.

Friedman, G.D., Siegelaub, A.B. and Seltzer, C.C. 1974. Cigarettes, alcohol, coffee and peptic ulcer. New Eng. J. Med. 290: 469-473.

Heath, C.W. 1958. Differences between smokers and non-smokers. Arch. Intern. Med. 101: 377-388.

Higgins, M.W., Kjelsberg, M. and Metzner, H. 1967. Characteristics of smokers and non-smokers in Tecumseh, Michigan. I. The distribution of smoking habits in persons and families and their relationship to social characteristics. Amer. J. Epidemiol. 86: 45-59.

Klauder, J.V. and Winkelman, N.W. 1928. Pellagra among chronic alcoholic addicts. J.A.M.A. 90: 364-369.

Knupfer, G. 1966. Some methodological problems in the epidemiology of alcoholic beverage usage: Definition of amounts of intake. Amer. J. Public Health 56: 237-242.

Lelbach, W.K. 1974. Organic pathology related to volume and pattern of alcohol use. IN *Researches in Alcohol and Drug Problems*. Eds. Gibbons, R.J., Israel, Y., Kalant, H., Popham, R.E., Schmidt. W. and Smart, R.G. Vol. 1, 93-198, John Wiley and Sons, Inc., New York.

Lolli, G., Serianni, E., Banissoni, F., Golder, G., Mariani, A., McCarthy, R.G. and Toner, M. 1952. The use of wine and other alcoholic beverages by a group of Italians and Americans of Italian extraction. Quart. J. Stud. Alc. 13: 27-48.

Lolli, G., Serianni, E., Golder, G., Balboni, C. and Mariani, A. 1953. Further observations on the use of wine and other alcoholic beverages by Italians and Americans of Italian extraction. Quart. J. Stud. Alc. 14: 395-405.

Luzzatto-Fegiz, P. and Lolli, G. 1957. The use of milk and wine in Italy. Quart. J. Stud. Alc. 18: 355-381.

Matarazzo, J.D. and Saslow, G. 1960. Psychological and related characteristics of smokers and non-smokers. Psychol. Bull. 57: 493-513.

Neville, J.N., Eagles, J.A., Samson, G. and Olson, R.E. 1968. Nutritional status of alcoholics. Amer. J. Clin. Nutr. 21: 1329-1340.

Olsen, A.Y. 1950. A study of dietary factors, alcoholic consumption, and laboratory findings in 100 patients with hepatic cirrhosis and 200 non-cirrhotic controls. Amer. J. Med. Sci. 220: 477-485.

Pequignot, G. 1963. Les enquêtes par interrogatoire permettent-elles de déterminer la frequence de l'étiologie alcoolique des cirrhoses due foie. Bull. Acad. Med. 1473-1475, 90-97.

Pequignot, G. and Cyrulnik, F. 1970. Chronic diseases due to over-consumption of alcoholic drinks (excepting neuropsychiatric pathology). *Internat. Encyclopedia of Pharmacol. and Therap.* Sec. 20, 2: 375-412, Pergamon Press, Oxford, England.

Register, U.D., Marsh, S.R., Thurston, C.T., Fields, B.J., Horning, M.C., Hardinge, M.G. and Sanchez, A. 1972. Influence of nutrients on intake of alcohol. J.A.D.A. 61: 159-162.

Roe, D.A. 1978. Physical Rehabilitation and Employment of AFDC Recipients. Final Report to U.S.D.L., Washington, D.C.

Solms, H. 1976. Alcoholism in Europe. Ann. New York Acad. Sci. 273: 24-32.

Spies, T.D. and DeWolf, H.F. 1933. Observations on the etiological relationship of severe alcoholism to pellagra. Amer. J. Med. Sci. 186: 521-527.

Texon, M. 1948. Medical aspects of an alcoholic service in a general hospital. New York Med. 4: 22-31.

Williams, R.J. 1953. Alcoholism as a nutritional problem. J. Clin. Nutr. 1: 32-36.

Williams, R.J., Berry, L.J. and Beerstecher, E., Jr. 1950. Genetotrophic diseases: Alcoholism. Texas Rep. Biol. Med. 8: 238-241.

5

Alcohol Consumption and Body Weight

In the public image, there are two kinds of alcoholics, the obese and the emaciated. The underweight alcoholic is not necessarily considered to represent an end stage of the fat alcoholic, but rather the two types are believed to represent different societal groups. Physicians, who are not specifically concerned with the care of alcoholics in alcoholism units, stress obesity as a sign of alcoholism, or rather suggest that unexplained fatness may indicate an excessive ingestion of ethanol. Bates (1965), in writing on the diagnosis of alcoholism, emphasizes demographic variables including unemployment, unmarried state, middle-age, habits including heavy smoking, heavy consumption of coffee, irregularities in eating pattern, irregularities in sleeping pattern, and a tendency to be immoderate in all things. This author defines alcoholism as a "overindulgence syndrome." He further states that "if a person is maintaining his weight, and the food he eats is low in calories . . . suspect addition of calories from alcohol." Other pointers to alcoholism cited by this author include a green tongue from chlorophyl lozenges, tatooing, bitten fingernails and fingers stained with tobacco. His image is of a man rather than a woman, though his definitions are not exclusive to the male. Ten years earlier a WHO technical report (1955) was devoted to the incidence of obesity among habitual heavy beer drinkers.

If we are to believe that obesity may be etiologically related to alcohol abuse, then relationships must be clearly defined. Following Bates' concept, it may be proposed that certain alcoholics, or heavy alcohol drinkers, not only drink more than they should, but also eat excessively. A modification of this idea is that drinkers may consume alcohol as an energy supplement to their accustomed diet.

CALORIC EXCESS FROM ALCOHOL AND FOOD

Consumption of alcohol calories may lead to caloric excess:

1. When drinkers frequently attend cocktail parties or other social occasions where snack food is also served.
2. When subjects under experimental conditions are deliberately invited to consume alcoholic beverages as an addition to their daily diet.
3. When it is the cultural norm to drink wine at or between meals.
4. When alcohol abusers are exposed to situational factors at work which encourage multiple eating and drinking occasions during the course of the day.

Bebb *et al.* (1971) (previously cited) investigated the effects of drinking on food consumption in 155 adults who were not considered to be alcoholics. In this study, one group consisted in 41 women and 32 men who had multiple sclerosis with varying degrees of disability. The other two groups who did not have multiple sclerosis consisted in 54 men who were employed in executive or managerial positions and 28 men who were taking part in a physical fitness program. It was found that as the percent of the total energy (calories) intake from alcohol increased, there was also a progressive increase in the average daily energy intakes. Among the subjects, weight changes were not related by the investigators to alcohol consumption. Indeed, it is the opinion of the present author that it would have been misleading to examine relationships between weight and alcohol consumption, since a subgroup of the total sample were suffering from a chronic disease which can, in itself, affect body weight.

In a Swedish study by Belfrage and coworkers, reported in 1973, alcohol was given daily for 5 weeks to healthy young men as light beer. Drinks were taken in four doses during the afternoon and evening, such that the total daily intake was 63 grams, which corresponded to about 16% of the daily energy intake reported. The intake of the beer induced a mean 17% increase in total energy intake, corresponding to that provided by the ethanol. Increases in body weight of 1-3 kg occurred during the period that the beer was given in seven out of the eight subjects studied.

The studies cited offer examples of circumstances in which intake of calories from alcoholic beverages is additive to food-calorie consumption. A Finnish study by Hasunen *et al.* (1977) shows that in certain groups of heavy alcohol consumers, food intake may actually be higher than in those who are more abstemious. In another study by

Tofler *et al.* (1969), it was found that among healthy employed middle-aged men the heaviest subjects consumed the greatest amount of alcohol, and in this group weight gain was correlated with both heavy current beer and total alcohol consumption.

BODY FATNESS AND ALCOHOL INTAKE

Relationships between body fatness and alcohol consumption differ according to the characteristics of the sample studied. D'Alonzo and Pell (1968) found that the proportion of heavy drinkers and controls who were more than 20% over their ideal body weights were similar, but more alcohol abusers were below their ideal weight than non-drinkers.

Myrhed (1974) studied 70 twin pairs in which the drinking habits of one member of the twin pair was different from the other. Both monozygous and dizygous twins were studied. Whereas no significant relationship was found between alcohol consumption and measures of body weight, the drinking member of the pairs had significantly larger triceps skinfold thickness, indicating a thicker layer of subcutaneous fat in this region.

Relationships between alcohol consumption and fatness cannot be dissociated from genetic or sociocultural factors which may influence body size and composition as well as intake of particular alcoholic beverages and foods.

In a report by Abdushelishvili (1976) from the USSR, indices of obesity in wine-making and drinking areas of East Georgia were shown to be higher than in Western Georgia where less wine is produced and drunk. There, differences in the incidence of obesity were found among rural population groups similarly engaged in semi-mechanized physical labor.

An investigation was undertaken by Klatsky and coworkers (1977) of people who took part in a multiphasic health checkup in the Oakland or San Francisco facilities of the Kaiser-Permanente Medical Care Program between July, 1964 and August, 1968. The sample consisted of 110,970 men and women between the ages of 15 and 79 years. The prevalence of drinking was heaviest in men and women between the ages of 20-29 years. Abstinence was more common among Orientals. Among the Caucasian males, total abstinence as well as heavy day drinking were most common in those with the lowest educational levels and with higher education, the proportion of non-drinkers was markedly decreased. This was also true among White women, though in this group, high daily alcohol intake did not vary with educational level. Both Black and Oriental men showed trends in alcohol consumption which were similar to those of the White women, and again, among these racial groups there was a relationship between educational level obtained and the number of people who were moderate drinkers. Among White males there was a slightly positive relationship between alcohol consumption and Quetelet's Index [weight/height^2] $\times$ 100 which was used as an index of adiposity. Among the Black males there was no significant relationship between alcohol consumption and Quetelet's Index. Among both Black and White women, the abstainers were the fattest groups. Among the Oriental subjects, there were no clear relationships between alcohol consumption and adiposity, either using Quetelet's Index or the Ponderal Index (height/^{3}weight).

The distribution of selected physical measurements and physiologic variables and the prevalence of certain diseases in smokers and non-smokers was studied by Higgins and Kjelsberg (1967). Cigarette smokers of both sexes, over the age of 20 years, weighed less than non-smokers of similar drinking habits. For women with similar smoking habits, non-drinkers were heavier than drinkers in all age subgroups over the age of 20 and these findings were similar among men under the age of 30. Above this age, male drinkers were heavier than non-drinkers. Women who neither smoked nor drank weighed most and those who smoked and drank weighed least. Men under the age of 40 weighed slightly more if they were non-smokers and non-drinkers and for the younger men, 20-29 years, those who smoked and drank were lighter. However, for men over the age of 40, current drinkers who were non-smokers, weighed most.

In the course of a study of relationships between alcohol intake and coronary risk factors in an Italian population group, Henze *et al.* (1977) found an inverse relationship between wine consumption and skinfold thickness (r=0.075, p<0.001). The sample group consisted in 2,588 men between the ages of 40-59 years who were included in the Italian section of the WHO Multifactor Preventive Trial of Coronary Heart Disease. Subjects were divided into 5 groups:

1. abstainers;
2. drinkers of less than ½ liter of wine per day;
3. drinkers of about ½ liter of wine per day;
4. those who drank about one liter/day; and
5. those who drank more than a liter of wine per day.

Recent anthropometric studies by the author (Roe, 1978), of two sample groups on public assistance in Upstate New York, included height/weight/age, arm muscle circumference, and triceps skinfold thickness measurements in non-drinkers, "social" drinkers and alcoholics so defined by the referring social agency and by corroborative data from a multiphasic health evaluation. Both sex and group differences were found, indicating a higher prevalence of obesity in women than in men($\Upsilon = .30$, p< .001, n=264). Alcoholics were more likely to be thin than fat (r = .14, p < .05, n =261). However, arm muscle circumference was not significantly different between drinking groups of either sex (Table 5.1).

TABLE 5.1 ANTHROPOMETRIC MEASUREMENTS OF NON–DRINKERS, DRINKERS, AND ALCOHOLICS IN LOW INCOME GROUPS*

Group	Mean Age	Skinfold Thickness mm	Age Specific** Minimum Skinfold Thickness Indicating Obesity (mm)	% Obese
Women				
Non-drinkers	36	27 (8-48)	30	41
Drinkers	34	26 (8-56)	30	32
Alcoholics	33	21 (10-45)	30	22
Controls	30	20 (6-71)	30	8
Men				
Non-drinkers	29	20 (6-38)	22	31
Drinkers	30	14 (4-43)	23	17
Alcoholics	32	14 (7-34)	23	16
Controls	28	11 (5-18)	22	0

*Downey, 1978
**Mayer, 1968

Among the women, the highest incidence of obesity was 41% in the non-drinkers. Female drinkers and alcoholics had obesity rates of 32% and 22% respectively. Men who did not drink had an obesity rate of 31%, whereas male drinkers and alcoholics had obesity rates of 17% and 10%. Obesity rates for a control group of age matched subjects, not on public assistance, showed an 8% prevalence in women and zero percent in men.

The major factors related to obesity in the female group, irrespective of drinking habits, was lack of physical activity. We are therefore led to the conclusion that the occurrence of obesity among non-drinkers, drinkers and alcoholics is related to sociocultural factors which influence activity as well as both eating and drinking habits. Interactions between socioeconomic status, drinking habit and obesity in women and men are illustrated in Fig. 5.1.

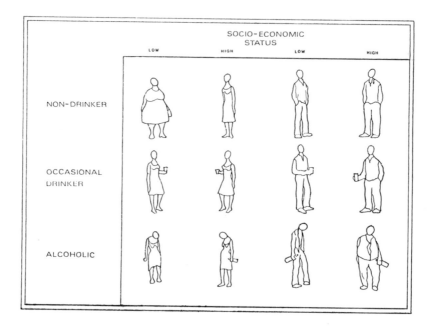

FIG. 5.1.   SEX CHARACTERISTICS, SOCIOECONOMIC STATUS, AND DRINKING
HABITS AS DETERMINANTS OF BODY WEIGHT.

ALCOHOL ABUSE AND WEIGHT LOSS

A metabolic explanation is offered by Pirola and Lieber (1976) for leanness among heavy drinkers. It is postulated that microsomal oxidation of ethanol in the liver and in other tissues is an energy wasting process so that when alcohol is consumed repeatedly, this factor could have quantitative significance in energy balance. Whereas evidence is presented to support this viewpoint, the alternate hypothesis that alcohol abuse may increase energy losses in the urine and feces has not been supported by human studies (Pirola and Lieber, 1972).

Clearly the Pirola-Lieber theory does not fully explain weight loss or wasting among alcoholics. Weight loss in the alcoholic and particularly in the binge-drinking alcoholic is determined by irregular eating habits and total or near total abstinence from food during and immediately after drinking bouts. Wasting is also secondary to the presence of alcoholic diseases including alcoholic hepatitis, cirrhosis and alcoholic myopathy. Wide excursions in body weight in alcoholics can be explained by periodic drinking alternated with enforced or voluntary abstinence as well as by the progression and/or remission of alcoholic disorders.

SELECTED REFERENCES

Abdushelishvili, G. 1976. The peculiarities of obesity frequency in the Georgian Republic, Proc. 10th. Internat. Congr. Nutrit. 1975, Kyoto, Japan, Victory-sha Press, pp. 263-264.

Bates, R.C. 1965. The diagnosis of alcoholism. Appl. Therap. 7: 466-469.

Bebb, H.T., Houser, H.B., Witschi, J.C., Littell, A.S. and Fuller, R.K. 1971. Calorie and nutrient contribution of alcoholic beverages to the usual diets of 155 adults. Amer. J. Clin. Nutr. 24: 1042-1052.

Belfrage, P.,Berg, B., Cronholm, T., D., Hagerstrand, I., Johansson, B., Nilsson-Ehle, P., Norden, G., Sjorvall, J. and Wiebe, T. 1973. Prolonged administration of ethanol to young healthy volunteers: Effects on biochemical, morphological and neurophysiological parameters. Acta Med. Scand. Suppl. 552: 5-44.

D'Alonzo, C.A. and Pell, S. 1968. Cardiovascular disease among problem drinkers. J. Occup. Med. 10: 865-872.

Downey, W.L. 1978. Nutrition and Alcoholism. Master's Degree Thesis. Ithaca, New York: Division of Nutritional Sciences, Cornell University.

Hasunen, K., Pekkarinen, M. and Nuutinen, O. 1977. Alcohol consumption and dietary intake of Finnish men. Nutr. Metab. 21, Suppl. 1: 132-133.

Henze, K., Bucci, A., Signoretti, P., Menotti, A. and Ricci, G. 1977. Alcohol intake at coronary risk factors in a population group in Rome. Nutrit. Metab. 21: suppl. 1, 157-159.

Higgins, M.W., and Kjelsberg, M. 1967. Characteristics of smokers and non-smokers in Tecumseh, Michigan II., Amer. J. Epidemiol. 86:60-77.

Klatsky, A.L., Friedman, G.D., Siegelaub, A.B. and Gerard, M.J. 1977. Alcohol consumption among white, black or oriental men and women: Kaiser-Permanente Multiphasic Health Examination data. Amer. J. Epidemiol. 105: 311-323.

Mayer, J. 1968. *Overweight: Causes, Cost and Control.* Englewood Cliffs, N.J. Prentice Hall, Inc.

Myrhed, M. 1974. Alcohol consumption in relation to factors associated with ischemic heart disease: A co-twin control study. Acta Med. Scand. Suppl. 567: 8-92.

Pirola, R.C. and Lieber, C.S. 1972. The energy cost of metabolism of drugs including ethanol. Pharmacology 7: 185-196.

Pirola, R.C. and Lieber, C.S. 1976. Hypothesis: Energy wastage in alcoholism and drug abuse: possible role of hepatic microsomal enzymes. Amer. J. Clin. Nutr. 29: 90-93.

Roe, D.A. 1978. Physical Rehabilitation and Employment of AFDC Recipients. Final Report to U.S.D.L., Washington, D.C.

Tofler, O.B., Saker, B.M., Rollo, K.A., Burvill, M.J. and Stenhouse, N. 1969. Electrocardiogram of the social drinker in Perth, Western Australia. Brit. Heart J. 31: 306-313.

WHO Technical Report. 1955. Obesity in Habitual Beer Drinkers, Ser. 94: 12.

6

Fetal Dysmaturity and the Alcoholic Woman

The ancients believed that drunkenness of the father leads to the birth of a retarded child. Aristotle further considered that foolish drunken women had similar children (Rolleston, 1927). The idea that intemperate parents may have undersized, malformed and mentally defective children has been a popular belief since early times, but particularly since the social evils of alcoholism have been recognized. In the 19th century Temperance workers subscribed to this belief, in order to encourage sobriety. At the same time, scientists who supported the idea that alcohol could damage the germ plasm, also allowed that alcoholism in one or both parents could be harmful to the child's development. In the first decade of the present century, several scientific inquiries were conducted to examine questions relating to the influence of parental alcoholism on the children. Reports of these investigations show evidence that drinking parents have drinking children; that the children of alcoholics exhibit physical defect; that the number of idiots and imbeciles born to alcoholic parents exceeds the number of similar children born to sober or temperate parents; and that the infants of alcoholics display retarded growth.

Professor Karl Pearson and Ethel Elderton of the Eugenics Laboratory of the University of London in 1910 sharply criticized all of these studies, both with respect to research design and data analysis. They considered that the claims of the investigators could not be substantiated by the data. Particularly, they disapproved of the use which had been made by Sir Victor Horsley of these studies to support his own temperance standpoint. The Pearson-Elderton critique ends on the note that associations between "extreme alcoholism" with defectiveness in the offspring could imply an association other than that

96

previously considered: that mentally defective and alcoholic parents have mentally defective offspring, and that the inheritance is of mental defectiveness and not of alcoholism as was suggested by the other investigators (MacNicholl, 1905; 1909; Laitinen, 1910; Madden, 1899; Bezzola, 1902; Pearson and Elderton, 1910).

Studies which are not cited by Pearson and Elderton but which belong to the same period and relate to the effects of parental alcoholism on the young are those by Sullivan (1900), who reported an increased incidence of stillbirths among the children of female alcoholics, and that of Ladrague (1901), who reported that the children of alcoholics are "small and sickly."

These reports all point up a serious deficiency of early studies of the prenatal effects of alcohol on the development and postnatal growth of a child. The attempt was made in most of the studies to answer too many questions which should properly have been posed separately, and then uniformly results of the studies were interpreted without insight into interacting or confounding variables.

Gordon Green (1974), in reviewing the early literature on relationships between parental alcoholism and child development, or the development of young animals, makes several pertinent comments. He states,

> These human and animal studies may be criticized on a variety of grounds. In some cases the authors had an axe to grind. In most, controls were lacking or inadequate. In short, little serious work had been done on a problem which may have existed since the year 8000 B.C. . . . The picture of alcoholic mothers is often complicated by additional variables: economic status, minority group status, nutritional status, prenatal care, anxiety and stress and others. Thus it is difficult to divide the factors and isolate the problems caused by the ethanol component.

Present concern is with the diet and nutrition of the alcoholic woman and to what extent this can explain retarded development and developmental anomalies found among the offspring of alcoholic women. However, before this subject can be approached, it is important to summarize established facts about alcohol and human development and to indicate gray areas where it is still not known whether it is alcohol or factors related to alcoholism which influence the children in alcoholic families.

THE INFLUENCE OF PARENTAL ALCOHOLISM ON THE DEVELOPMENT AND SURVIVAL OF CHILDREN

The first serious study of the effects of parental alcoholism on the development, health and survival of offspring was that conducted by Elderton and Pearson (1910a). The aim of these studies was to investigate effects of parental alcoholism, that is, alcoholism in the mother or father, on the development and survival of the children. They did not examine any effects on the children of the mother drinking excessively during pregnancy. The sample populations utilized consisted in children attending special schools in Manchester, England, and children attending an elementary school in Edinburgh, Scotland. In both instances the children tended to come from low income families, though in the case of the Edinburgh sample, there was an admixture of children from problem homes and those from homes that were "substantially comfortable." A selection bias occurred with respect to the Manchester sample, in that in the families studied at least one child was mentally defective. Important findings included a higher death rate among the offspring of alcoholic than among the offspring of sober parents. It was found that these differences were more marked in the case of the mother being alcoholic than in the case of the father. Interestingly, the authors considered that this differential death rate could, in large part, be explained by accidents and gross carelessness on the part of the parents, and that it could only be explained to a minor extent by a toxic effect of the alcohol on the offspring. The heights and weights of the children, corrected for age, were slightly greater in the children of sober parents. When certain health parameters were examined, it was found that the general health of the children of the alcoholic parents appeared to be slightly better than the health of the children of sober parents, and this was explained through the unproven hypothesis that there was a survival of the fittest or that the higher death rate of the children of alcoholic parents may leave the fitter to survive. There was no evidence from this study that parental alcoholism led to mental defect in the offspring. No strong relationship was found between the intelligence, physique or disease of the offspring and parental alcoholism in any of the categories investigated.

Haggard and Jellinek (1942) examined the outcome of gestation in alcoholic mothers; figures being taken from England, France, Finland, and Austria. Conclusions were that 1) the number of children in alcoholic families was greater; 2) alcoholic mothers have more spontaneous abortions; and 3) alcoholic mothers have a high infant death rate—the figure given being almost twice that of non-alcoholic mothers.

Roe (1945) commented on the high infant mortality among the children of alcoholics and the finding that epilepsy, idiocy and psychosis are common among these children. Christiaens *et al.* (1960) discussed the increased incidence of prematurity among children of alcoholics and also that these children showed low heights and weights at follow-up.

Returning to the studies by Roe, she has suggested that "the higher mortality among the offspring of alcoholics can be adequately explained by the neglect and poor care to which they are subject, and that there is no necessity to hypothesize poor germ plasm as an explanation." Her studies were of adults of alcoholic and non-alcoholic parentage who had been placed in foster homes in childhood. She found that the offspring of the normal parentage group received more schooling and reached higher levels of achievement than the children of alcoholics. Whereas it was considered conceivable that this difference could relate to the value placed on education by the foster parents, it was considered more likely, from various lines of evidence, that the children of alcoholics were less able to avail themselves of educational possibilities or to develop skills, because they were less intelligent. There were no inebriates in the foster children from either group.

FETAL DYSMATURITY AND THE FETAL ALCOHOL SYNDROME

It is difficult to document when fetal dysmaturity was first recorded in the offspring of mothers given to alcohol abuse during their pregnancies. Symposia and texts on fetal dysmaturity up to 1973 make no direct reference to maternal alcoholism as a cause. However, among case histories of dysmature infants described by Ounsted and Ounsted (1973), case 21 strongly suggests the syndrome which has now been entitled the fetal alcohol syndrome.

Beargie *et al.* (1970) described a retrospective investigation of low birth weight infants seen at the University of Kentucky Medical Center. The study population consisted in 45 infants of 42 mothers. Three of the mothers were chronic alcoholics. The authors found out that these three women were not only drinking heavily during pregnancy, but often were without food for long periods of time. Their infants were markedly wasted at the time of birth and two of them showed postnatal growth retardation at follow-up. In this study population as a whole, those infants who had undergone the longest prenatal insult were most undergrown and least well developed at the time of follow-up examinations when the children were between the ages of 13 and 53 months.

Lemoine *et al.* (1967) are considered the first authors to have described what we now call the fetal alcohol syndrome. They reported on a series of 127 children of chronic alcoholics from 69 families in Nantes, France. Four major findings were common to the study population, viz. 1) peculiar facies, 2) growth retardation, 3) increased frequency of malformations, and 4) psychomotor problems.

In 1972, Ulleland reported observations on six infants seen at the University of Washington's Harbor View Medical Center, whose mothers were all alcoholic. The infants were small-for-dates, with a birth weight below the tenth percentile, and their postnatal growth and development were retarded. The characteristics of these infants, and particularly their failure to thrive despite special attention to feeding, prompted investigation of other low birth weight infants who had been delivered at the Harbor View Medical Center. During an 18 month period of chart review, 1,594 babies were delivered at the hospital, of whom 47 or 2.9%, were small-for-dates. Thirty seven, or 2.3% of these infants, were offspring of non-alcoholic mothers, whereas 10 of the 12 infants born to alcoholic mothers showed evidence of prenatal growth retardation. The alcoholic mothers, as might be anticipated, exhibited several characteristics which could contribute to the growth retardation of their children. Parity was high. Only four of the mothers had received any prenatal care. Two of the mothers were heavy smokers. Three showed evidence of cirrhosis on liver biopsy. Diet history indicated that two of the mothers had moderate to severe deficiencies pertaining to energy or protein intake during their pregnancies. Three of them admitted to taking 25% or more of their daily energy intake as alcohol. Biochemical assessment of nutritional status did not reveal severe deficiencies. However, data given are incomplete in this respect. It is tempting to consider from this study that pre and postnatal growth retardation in the infants of alcoholic women may be multifactorial and not only related to the toxic effect of the alcohol, but also to fetal malnutrition.

In 1973 Jones *et al.* described a syndrome of prenatal growth deficiency and multi-system defects followed by postnatal growth retardation in infants whose mothers were given to alcohol abuse. Among eight unrelated children, defects were variable in extent, system of involvement and severity. Cranio-facial, limb and cardiovascular abnormalities were found in these children. Six of the eight children showed aberrant palmar creases. From the nutritional standpoint, it is important to note that, despite the fact that adequate caloric intake was recorded, catch-up growth did not occur in at least six of the children during hospitalization for "failure to thrive." The fact that, in these children, prenatal growth retardation affected length more than weight is suggested as an argument against maternal undernutrition or malnutrition as a cause of the infant's retarded development. In late dysmaturity, due to maternal undernutrition in the third trimester of pregnancy, infants tend to be of normal length but are variably underweight.

Further study of the offspring of alcoholic women by this group indicated a prenatal mortality of 17%. Prenatal growth deficiency, postnatal growth retardation, and borderline to moderate mental deficiency were common features among offspring of alcoholic women. It is emphasized that "deficient intellectual performance" was the most frequent problem noted in the surviving children, usually accompanied by diminished head circumference. According to these authors, therapeutic abortion should be considered in women subject to alcohol abuse during pregnancy. Such action would be justified because of the permanent physical and mental damage to so many of these children (Jones et al., 1974).

Since 1973 the syndrome of pre and postnatal growth retardation associated with developmental defects and variable degrees of mental retardation in the children of alcoholic women has been termed "the fetal alcohol syndrome." In 1975 Jones and Smith calculated that the most common manifestations of the syndrome included prenatal growth deficiency, postnatal growth deficiency, developmental delay, short palpebral fissures, microcephaly, and fine motor dysfunction. Hanson et al. (1976) mention the occurrence of developmental anomalies in children with the fetal alcohol syndrome including microphthalmos, cataract, abnormal retinal pigmentation, cardiac defects, joint and skeletal anomalies, diaphragmatic defects, cleft palate, hemangiomata and genital anomalies.

Discussion of the etiology of the fetal alcohol syndrome by Jones and Smith (1975) has suggested a direct toxic effect of ethanol on fetal tissues. Other etiological possibilities which have been considered by these authors include toxic effects of acetaldehyde, or of some unknown congener in the alcoholic beverage that was consumed. The suggestion that the developmental defects and growth retardation could be due to maternal malnutrition is considered to be highly unlikely.

Mulvihill et al. (1975) have reported on the characteristics of the fetal alcohol syndrome among infants observed in the department of pediatrics at the Johns Hopkins University School of Medicine. Important points made by these authors include the long duration of the maternal alcoholism and the fact that the nature of the alcohol or alcohol mixture consumed did not appear to influence the outcome. Poor eating habits, pregnancy anemia, heavy smoking, and other substance abuse are mentioned in the mothers of children with the fetal alcohol syndrome from this center. It was emphasized that several interactive factors may influence the outcome of gestation in an alcoholic. Alcohol is considered as the teratogen, but perhaps not the only teratogen in alcoholic beverages; other compounds such as aldehydes and heavy metals which can cross the placenta could also damage the fetus. Inadequate nutrition of the mother is also considered as a possible etiological factor by these workers. Fetal alcohol syndrome has been observed in twins and also in siblings; these observations being explained by the persistent exposure of the developing fetus to the causal agent (Christoffel and Salafsky, 1975).

Smith *et al.* (1976) indicate that in the offspring of women who are chronic alcoholics, about one-third have the fetal alcohol syndrome and almost a half have various degrees of mental deficiency. It is suggested that the epidemiology of the syndrome would follow the incidence of chronic alcoholism in women. The facies of children with fetal alcohol syndrome has been accurately described and pictured in several papers. Cranio-facial abnormalities include short palpebral fissures, epicanthic folds, ptosis, maxillary hypoplasia, cleft palate and micrognathia. Indeed, to the writer, the syndrome is particularly suggested by the combination of short palpebral fissure and ptosis, as well as more recently described aberrant features of the face, including upturned nostrils and a carp-like mouth (Jones *et al.*, 1976) (Figure 6.1).

The precise causation of the fetal alcohol syndrome is not known. Recently Mulvihill and Yeager (1977) pointed out that "the risk of a fetus being affected may be directly related to the amount of alcohol it is exposed to, that the actual dose and duration of exposure required are unknown."

However, in a 1974 study reported by Ouellette *et al.* (1977), questionnaires were administered to 633 women in prenatal care at the Boston City Hospital. Information was obtained on food intake, using a 24 hour recall method. The present and past intake of alcohol and drugs, as well as smoking habits, were determined. Dietary analysis included an assessment of the adequacy of nine nutrients in relation to the Recommended Dietary Allowances for women from 20-30 years of age. The volume and frequency of monthly alcohol intakes were calculated and drinking patterns were classified, so that patients could be divided into three groups. Group 1 consisted of 326 women (52%) who drank less than once a month, these women being termed abstinent or rare drinkers. Group 2 were those women composing 39% of the sample who

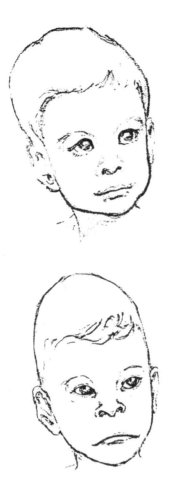

FIG. 6.1 FACIAL APPEARANCE OF CHILD BELOW WITH
"FETAL ALCOHOL SYNDROME" AND NORMAL CHILD ABOVE.

drank more than once a month but did not meet the criteria imposed for heavy drinkers and Group 3, the heavy drinkers, constituting 9% of the sample, were women who consumed five or more drinks on occasion and had a consistent daily intake of more than 45 ml of absolute alcohol. Developmental examination of the infants was carried out on the second or third day after delivery. Dietary assessment did not indicate significant differences in nutrient intake between the three groups of women. However, diet recall may be misleading, particularly in alcoholics. Heavy drinkers were also heavy smokers. Significant differences between groups were found with respect to incidence of malformations and growth abnormalities in the offspring, such that at neonatal examination, 71% of the offspring of heavy drinkers, 45% of the offspring of light drinkers, and 36% of the rare drinkers were abnormal by the criteria imposed. Birth weight and length was lower in the infants of heavy drinkers and congenital anomalies were more frequent. The ability to suck was also reduced in babies in this group. The authors comment that whereas heavy drinking during the first trimester may have an adverse effect on fetal development, heavy drinking in the last trimester is likely to impair fetal nutrition.

EXPERIMENTAL DATA ON FETAL DISPOSITION OF ETHANOL AND THE FETAL ALCOHOL SYNDROME

Basic information on the transplacental passage of ethanol and its fetal metabolism justifies the hypothesis that ethanol is the primary toxic agent. The transplacental transfer of ethanol has been studied in pregnant women, but no gradient has been established between maternal and fetal blood levels after ethanol infusion. At birth, ethanol concentrations have been found to be similar in the maternal and infant circulations. The rate of elimination of ethanol is slow in fetal monkeys and hamsters, as well as human neonates. In fetal mammalian livers, in contrast to mature livers of animals of the same species, there is a reduced activity of alcohol dehydrogenase, which accounts for differential rates of alcohol metabolism (Mirkin and Singh, 1976; Idanpään-Heikkilä et al., 1972; Idanpään-Heikkilä et al., 1971; Pikkarainen and Räihä, 1967).

Rawat (1976) has shown that in the rat, the appearance of alcohol dehydrogenase in the fetal liver controls hepatic ethanol oxidation capacity, but, however, changes in the neonatal liver redox state appearing immediately after birth do not influence activity of this enzyme. Metabolites and nutrients having a positive or accelerating effect on hepatic ethanol oxidation rate include pyruvates in the fetal as well as neonatal liver, and fructose and alanine in the neonatal liver, but not in the fetal liver.

While caution must be exercised in extrapolating these data to human fetuses or infants, these studies by Rawat suggest two inferences: that the fetus is at the biochemical disadvantage with respect to alcohol detoxication, and that nutrients or biochemical metabolites of nutrients which may be more or less available to the infant play a role in ethanol metabolism.

Our most recent knowledge of the causal factors determining the development of the fetal alcohol syndrome come from the studies by Chernoff (1977) on the effects of alcohol on the fetal mouse. This investigator maintained CBA/J and C3H pregnant mice on liquid diets consisting in Metrecal with ethanol for the experimental groups and Metrecal without ethanol for the controls. The diets were the complete feed for the mice for 30 days before and throughout gestation. The dams were killed on the 18th day of gestation, and the offspring were examined for malformations. In both strains of mice, the fetal resorption rate increased with an increasing intake of ethanol derived calories, but the CBA strain were more sensitive to ethanol intake, or possibly to deprivation of other nutrients. It should be noted that daily energy intakes of the mice of both strains decreased with an increased consumption of ethanol derived calories and with increased blood ethanol levels. Reduction in fetal weight, deficient ossification of the occiput, and certain neural anomalies were found in mice on low ethanol diets and with the higher ethanol intake other malformations were detected, more particularly cardiac defects.

While this study is a major step forward in investigation of the fetal alcohol syndrome, since it demonstrates that the fetal alcohol syndrome or a similar pathology can be induced in the mouse, it has not been shown precisely that ethanol per se is teratogenic. Further investigations are required to show whether ethanol alone is teratogenic, or whether there is a synergistic or additive effect of ethanol and fetal malnutrition in the production of the fetal alcohol syndrome either in the animal model or in human subjects. If, as was shown in these experiments in the mouse, food intake by the dam is reduced by substitution of ethanol calories, then also the intakes of other nutrients will be reduced. In experimental animals, specific nutrient deficiencies have been associated both with retarded prenatal development and the induction of malformations. Hurley and Mutch (1973) showed that when rats were fed a zinc deficient diet between days 6 and 14 of pregnancy, they gave birth to offspring with reduced body weight and a high incidence of congenital malformations. Maternal pyridoxine deficiency in the rat has also been associated with impairment in cellular growth and development of the progeny (Moon and Kirksey, 1973).

Folate deficiency in pregnant rats during the period of embryogenesis has been associated with multiple malformations as well as early fetal death and resorption. Several of the defects associated with folate deficiency are similar to those associated with the experimental fetal alcohol syndrome including defects of the cardiovascular system and the nervous system (Cooper et al., 1970).

Complex drug-nutrient interrelationships may have etiological significance in the fetal alcohol syndrome. In the rat, zinc deficiency impairs conversion of retinol to retinal as well as the catabolism of ethanol, because it reduces activity of alcohol dehydrogenase (Huber and Gershoff, 1975).

COMMENTS ON THE ENVIRONMENTAL ADVERSITY OF THE ALCOHOLIC WOMAN'S CHILD

In the present state of our knowledge, it seems clear that retardation in physical and mental development of the offspring of female alcoholics who drink during pregnancy is related to the fetal alcohol syndrome. Since in the animal model the effects of ethanol feeding with the possible interaction of nutrient depletion gave rise to a symptom complex resembling the fetal alcohol syndrome in human subjects, it is no longer justifiable to infer that such variables as maternal smoking could be influential in that condition. However, the birth of small-for-dates infants without evidence of malformation to alcoholic mothers may well also be associated with such factors as maternal smoking habits and maternal malnutrition. Smoking has an adverse effect on fetal growth rates. However, since the degree of fetal growth retardation is not directly related to the number of cigarettes that are smoked, it has been suggested by Ounsted and Ounsted (1973) that other habits of smokers may contribute to the observed growth retardation. Alcohol use has been associated strongly with cigarette smoking by Klatsky et al. (1977) and by other authors previously cited, indicating that smoking per se or diminished maternal food intake, associated with smoking, may influence the degree of dysmaturity in the offspring of alcoholics at birth.

SELECTED REFERENCES

Beargie, R.A., James, V.L., and Greene, J.W. 1970. Growth and development of small-for-date newborns. Pediat. Clin. N. America 17: 159-167.

Bezzola, A. 1902. Statistische Untersuchungen uber die Rolle des Alkohols bei der Ensthung des uriginaren Schwachsinns. Proc. 8th Internat. Congress on Alcoholism. Vienna, April 1901, Leipzig and Vienna Publ. p. 109-111.

Chernoff, G.F. 1977. The fetal alcohol syndrome in mice: An animal model. Teratology 15: 223-230.

Christiaens, L., Mizon, J.P. and Delmarle, G. 1960. On the descendants of alcoholics. Ann. Pediat. 36: 37-42.

Christoffel, K.K. and Salafsky, I. 1975. Fetal alcohol syndrome in dizygotic twins. J. Pediat. 87: 963-967.

Cooper, B.A., Cantlie, G.S.D. and Brunton, L. 1970. The case for folic acid supplements during pregnancy. Amer. J. Clin. Nutr. 23: 848-854.

Elderton, E.M. and Pearson, K. 1910. A first study of the influence of parental alcoholism on the physique and ability of the offspring. Eugenics Lab Mem. X: Univ. London, Dulau and Co. Ltd., London.

Gordon Green, H. 1974. Infants of alcoholic mothers. Amer. J. Obstet. Gynecol. 118: 713-716.

Haggard, H.W. and Jellinek, E.M. 1942. Alcohol Explored. Doubleday, Doran & Co., Ltd., Garden City, N.J..

Hanson, J.W., Jones, K.L. and Smith, D.W. 1976. Fetal alcohol syndrome. J. Amer. Med. Assoc. 235: 1458-1460.

Huber, A.M. and Gershoff, S.N. 1975. Effects of zinc deficiency on the oxidation of retinol and ethanol in rats. J. Nutr. 105: 1486-1490.

Hurley, L.S. and Mutch, P.B. 1973. Prenatal and postnatal development after transitory gestational zinc deficiency in rats. J. Nutr. 103: 649-656.

Idanpään-Heikkilä, J., Fritchie, G.E., Ho, B.T. and McIssac, W.M. 1971. Placental transfer of C^{14}-ethanol. Am. J. Obstet. Gynecol. 110: 426-428.

Idanpään-Heikkilä, J., Jouppilla, P., Akerblom, H.K., Isoaho, R., Kauppila, E., and Koivisto, M. 1972. Elimination and metabolic effects of ethanol in mother, fetus and newborn infant. Amer. J. Obstet. Gynecol. 112: 387-393.

Jones, K.L. and Smith, D.W. 1975. The fetal alcohol syndrome: Teratology 12: 1-10.

Jones, K.L., Smith, D.W. and Hanson, J.W. 1976. The fetal alcohol syndrome: Clinical delineation. Ann. N.Y. Acad. Sci. 273: 130-137.

Jones, K.L., Smith, D.W., Streissguth, A.P. and Myrianthopoulos, N.C. 1974. Outcome in offspring of chronic alcoholic women. Lancet 1: 1076-1078.

Jones, K.L., Smith, D.W., Ulelland, C.N. and Striessguth, A.P. 1973. Pattern of malformation in offspring of chronic alcoholic mothers. Lancet 1: 1267-1271.

Klatsky, A.L., Friedman, G.D., Siegelaub, A.B. and Gerard, M.J. 1977. Alcohol consumption among white, black, or oriental men and women: Kaiser-Permanente multiphase health examination data. Amer. J. Epidemiol. 105: 311-323.

Ladrague, P. 1901. Alcoholisme et Enfants. Steinheil, Paris.

Laitinen, T. 1910. Der Einfluss des Alkohols auf die Nach Kammenschaft des menschen. Internat. Monat. Z. Erforsch. d Alkoholismus. Basel, xx, pp. 193-198.

Lemoine, P.H., Harousseau, H., Borteyru, J.P. and Menuet, J.C. 1967. Les enfants de parents alcoholiques: Anomalies observeés a propos de 127 cas. Arc. Fr. Pédiat. 25: 830-832.

MacNicholl, T.A. 1905. A study of the effects of alcohol on school children. Med. Temp. Rev. 8: 247-249.

MacNicholl, T.A. 1909. Alcohol and heredity. Med. Temp. Rev. 12: 53-56.

Madden, J. 1899. Shall We Drink Wine. Owen and Weihbrecht Co., Milwaukee, 103-116.

Mirkin, B.L. and Singh, S. 1976. Placental transfer of pharmacologically active molecules. IN *Perinatal Pharmacology and Therapeutics.* Ed. Mirkin, B.L. Academic Press, New York, San Francisco, London. 48-49.

Moon, W.Y. and Kirskey, A. 1973. Cellular growth during prenatal and early postnatal periods in progeny of pyridoxine-deficient rats. J. Nutr. 103: 123-133.

Mulvihill, J.J. and Yeager, A.M. 1977. Fetal alcohol syndrome. Teratology 13: 345-348.

Mulvihill, J.J., Klimas, J.T., Stokes, D.C. and Risenberg, H.M. 1976. Fetal alcohol syndrome: Seven new cases. Amer. J. Obstet. Gynecol. 125: 937-941.

Ouellette, E.M., Rosett, H.L., Rosman, N.P., and Weiner, L. 1977. Adverse effects on offspring of maternal alcohol abuse during pregnancy. New Eng. J. Med. 297: 528-530.

Ounsted, M. and Ounsted, C. 1973. On Fetal Growth Rates (Its Variations and Their Consequences). IN *Clinics in Developmental Medicine 46*: Spastics International Med. Publ., London, Heinemann Med. Books Ltd., Philadelphia,J. B. Lippincott Co., p. 45-47; 164.

Pearson, K. and Elderton, E.M. 1910. A second study of the influence of parenteral alcoholism on the physique and ability of the offspring. Eugen. Lab. Mem. XIII, Univ. London, Dulau and Co., Ltd., London.

Pikkarainen, P.H. and Räihä, M.C. 1967. Development of alcohol dehydrogenase activity in the human liver. Pediat. Res. 1: 165-168.

Rawat, A.K. 1976. Effect of maternal ethanol consumption on fetal hepatic metabolism in the rat. IN Work in Progress on Alcoholism. Ann. N.Y. Acad. Sci. 273: 175-187.

Roe, A. 1945. The adult adjustment of children of alcoholic parents raised in foster homes. Quart. J. Stud. Alcohol 5: 378-393.

Rolleston, J.D. 1927. Alcoholism in classical antiquity. Brit. J. Inebriety 24: 101-120.

Smith, D.W., Jones, K.L. and Hanson, J.W. 1976. Perspectives on the cause and frequency of fetal alcohol syndrome. IN Work in Progress on Alcoholism. Ann. N.Y. Acad. Sci. 273: 138-139.

Sullivan, W.C. 1900. The children of the female drunkard. Med. Temp. Rev. 3: 72.

Ulelland, C.N. 1972. The offspring of alcoholic mothers. Ann. N.Y. Acad. Sci. 197: 167-169.

7

Effects of Alcohol on Nutrient Availability

Heavy ethanol ingestion has a direct toxic effect on the intestinal tract and more particularly on the small intestine. This adverse effect of ethanol occurs independently of alcohol related diseases, such as alcoholic pancreatitis and alcoholic liver disease, which can also cause maldigestion and malabsorption. The acute toxic effects of ethanol on the small intestine are manifest both during the period of intoxication, or active alcohol abuse, and during the immediate withdrawal period. Periods of cramping abdominal pain and diarrhea are usually associated with binge drinking in alcoholics. Studies in laboratory rats and in recently drinking alcoholics have indicated that these symptoms have a multifactorial etiology (Dinoso et al., 1971). Two causes of diarrhea currently most favored are alcohol induced disaccharidase deficiency, causing lactose intolerance, and alcohol-induced impairment in the absorption of water and electrolytes from the small intestine.

DISACCHARIDASE DEFICIENCY IN ALCOHOLICS

Inhibition of intestinal disaccharidase activity has been produced in laboratory rats by alcohol administration. Rats receiving high enough doses of alcohol to induce disaccharidase "deficiency" also show microscopic evidence of intestinal epithelial damage (Baraona et al., 1974). Since the intestinal disaccharidases are "packaged" along the brush border of the small intestine, and particularly in the jejunum, it is not difficult to understand why these enzymes should be inhibited either when the luminal contents contain ethanol or when ultrastructural changes occur in the brush border, as has been demonstrated following ingestion of alcohol (Rubin et al., 1972). Acute and chronic effects of ethanol on the small intestine have been differentiated by Baraona *et al.* (1974), with laboratory rats as the animal model. Acute damage to this part of the gastrointestinal tract was induced by intragastric administration of ethanol. Rats, in which effects of chronic alcohol administration was to be evaluated, received an ethanol-containing diet in which the concentration of ethanol was gradually increased to reach the maximal level of 5 g/100 ml then on the fifth day. The total duration of feeding the alcohol-containing diet was 3-4 weeks. Morphological assessments of the small intestine were made, both in the rats given alcohol by stomach tube on an acute basis, and in those accustomed to the alcohol-containing diet. Oxygen consumption was also measured in jejunal rings, and incubated in a Krebs-Ringer phosphate buffer (pH 7.4), containing 20 mM glucose. Enzyme assays on jejunal and ileal samples included determinations of lactase, sucrase, and alkaline phosphatase. Intragastric ethanol produced hemorrhagic lesions and small areas of necrosis in the stomach and similar but smaller hemorrhages in the intestinal mucosa. In some intestinal areas the petecchial hemorrages were, however, confluent. The most severe changes occurred in the tips of the villi which lost their epithelium and were covered with cellular debris. The intestinal lesions were concentrated in the first few centimeters of the duodenum and the jejunum and lessened in the more distal portions of the small intestine. The degree and extent of the acute lesions in the intestine induced by ethanol varied with the concentration. Chronic feeding of ethanol-containing diets did not produce hemorrhagic lesions but caused a reduction in the length of the jejunal villi and an increased epithelial cell count in the intestinal crypts.

The acute ethanol administration decreased the activity of the jejunal lactase and thymidine kinase. The alcohol-containing diet fed on a chronic basis also reduced the activity of these jejunal enzymes and this occurred whether the ethanol was isocalorically replacing carbohydrate or fat in the diet.

Among drinkers of Pilsner beers, it has been shown that intestinal activities of maltase and sucrase are reduced in intestinal biopsies, despite the fact that these drinks have a high maltose content, and it is known that maltose alone can enhance the activity of maltase (Madzarovova-Nohejlova, 1971). Perlow *et al.* (1977) studied the lactase and sucrase activities in jejunal biopsies from alcoholic and non-alcoholic men who were either American Blacks or Whites of Northern-European origin. If sucrase activity was measured within ten days of alcohol withdrawal, it was found to be decreased by 33% in the alcoholics. Negligible lactase activity was found in 100% of the Black and 20% of the White alcoholics, but only in 50% of the Black, and in none of the White, control subjects. After two weeks of alcohol withdrawal, increases were found in the levels of both disaccharidase activities in the intestinal epithelium. When lactose was administered, there was a lower blood-glucose concentration and a higher incidence of abdominal symptoms in the alcoholics, particularly those who were American Blacks. The authors consider that, since symptomatic lactose intolerance was found among the alcoholics, particularly those who were Black, impairment of lactose absorption must have been extensive. We interpret this to mean that lactose reached the large intestine, where it was fermented by the microflora with the production of lactic acid, causing the observed alcoholic diarrhea and a dumping-like syndrome. A further suggestion has been made that milk intolerance may become symptomatic when alcohol is drunk to excess in those who have genetically determined low levels of lactase in the intestine (Perlow *et al.*, 1977).

EFFECTS OF ETHANOL ON INTESTINAL ABSORPTIVE FUNCTION

In men and women who are alcoholics, acute ingestion of alcohol results in a drug-induced malabsorption syndrome. Impairment of D-xylose absorption has been demonstrated in chronic alcoholic patients with minimal liver disease who have been recently drinking (Mezey, 1975). Recovery of D-xylose absorption has been observed in chronic alcoholics after admission to hospital when they are receiving the diet of the institution, even when they continue to consume ethanol (Mezey *et al.*, 1970; Halsted *et al.*, 1971). Mezey (1975) has suggested that folacin deficiency resulting from ethanol abuse as well as dietary folacin deficiency, could cause intestinal malabsorption, which is reversed by higher folacin intake. Whereas Mezey also found steatorrhea in 33% of 42 chronic alcoholic patients on admission to hospital, this sign of malabsorption also disappeared when these patients were given an adequate diet, whether or not they were also receiving alcoholic beverages.

Ethanol has been shown to have an inhibitory effect on the active transport and absorption of nutrients. Using everted sacs of rat intestine, Israel *et al.* (1968) showed that ethanol significantly reduced the active transport of L-phenylalanine with concentrations between 0.5 - 2.0%. At the latter concentration of ethanol, active transport of L-methionine was abolished. *In vivo*, when ethanol was given to rats at a dosage of 250mg/100 gm body weight orally, the intestinal absorption of L-phenylalanine was reduced by 50%.

Ethanol diminishes the absorption of sodium chloride and water from the small intestine. Krasner *et al.* (1976b) came to this conclusion after investigating ten patients with chronic alcoholism who had several tests performed to ascertain whether or not malabsorption was present. The absorption of water and electrolytes from the jejunum was studied in this group using a triple-lumen tube perfusion system. The authors suggest that in patients in whom binge drinking is superimposed on chronic alcoholism, there is a functional impairment of electrolyte and water absorption. It is further postulated that some of the nutritional deficiencies which are prevalent in such patients, as well as gastrointestinal symptoms, may arise because of malabsorption. Among the cases described by Krasner et al., D-xylose absorption was decreased in a third of the patients.

Decreased absorption of micellar long-chain fatty acids has also been demonstrated in alcoholic patients. Malagelada *et al.* (1974) made this finding in ten alcoholics with documented cirrhosis, after they were admitted to a metabolic ward and placed on a bland hospital diet. Alcohol ingestion was stopped at the time of their hospital admission, which was six weeks prior to the study. No evidence was obtained to indicate that medium chain fatty acids were similarly malabsorbed. The question which remains unanswered is whether the impairment and absorption of long-chain fatty acids was related to hepatic dysfunction present in these patients, or whether it is a direct toxic effect of ethanol on the small intestine.

Whereas, in rats, it has been shown that ethanol does not delay fat absorption when given at relatively low dosage (2 gm/kg body weight), at higher dosages (greater than 3 gm of ethanol/kg body weight), delayed fat absorption is found (Barboriak and Meade, 1969). Whereas reduced exocrine function of the pancreas may explain in part ethanol-associated malabsorption of macronutrients, this would not explain reduced absorption of electrolytes in water, nor would it explain amino acid malabsorption (Sardesai and Orten, 1968).

Studies of effects of alcohol on the active transport of nutrients have been carried out. Krasner *et al.* (1976a) investigated ATP levels and ATPase activities in ethanol-treated guinea pig jejunum. ATP concentrations were significantly reduced in these ethanol-exposed jejunal segments, as compared to control portions of the guinea pig jejunum, which were exposed to Krebs' solution. No effect of ethanol was found on ATPase activity in these experiments. In further chronic studies of the effects of alcohol on the guinea pig intestine *in vivo*, ethanol was not found to affect either ATP levels or ATPase activity. Investigators have concluded that the effects of ethanol on the absorption of at least some water-soluble nutrients is due to the actual presence of the ethanol in the intestine, rather than some longer-term effect on mucosal function. While this is an interesting hypothesis, we would like to see further work to indicate or pinpoint effects of ethanol on active transport mechanisms. A recent editorial has emphasized that malabsorption in the alcoholic may be due to pathological changes which are induced in the intestine—an opinion with which we concur (Editorial, Nutr. Rev., 1977).

Folacin deficiency is prevalent in the chronic alcoholic, and as previously indicated, may arise from deficient intake, malabsorption, or an impaired utilization or hyperexcretion of folacin. It was shown by Hermos *et al.* (1972) that there are specific histological changes of folacin deficiency which can be demonstrated in the intestinal mucosa in alcoholics. These investigators obtained bone marrow aspirates, and peroral duodenojejunal biopsies on 21 occasions from 11 patients with chronic alcoholism and folacin deficiency. Although a statement is made that these patients, all of them men, had been "drinking heavily and eating poorly before admission," no detail is given with respect to their diets. The folacin deficiency was established in these patients by the finding of bone marrow megaloblastosis, a serum folacin level in the low or deficient range, and a normal serum vitamin B_{12} level. Associated, alcohol-related, diseases were present in several of the patients including cirrhosis and acute pancreatitis. There were seven control subjects who were considered to be healthy and who were not alcoholics. The significant histological abnormalities in the initial intestinal biopsies of three of the patients who had severe bone marrow megaloblastosis, included shortening of the villi, reduction in the thickness of the intestinal mucosa, increased cellularity of the lamina propria, and most importantly, megaloblastic changes in the epithelial cells of the villi. In two patients, effects of ethanol ingestion (24-32 oz. of 86-proof commercial whiskey, 234-312 g/day of ethanol) was studied with respect to effects on the bone marrow and the intestine. One of the patients also received folic acid while being given alcohol at the level mentioned above. Three patients were given pharmacologic doses of folic acid after hospital admission without any further alcohol. The two alcoholics who were given large quantities of alcohol, were reported as being well nourished prior to this time. While they received alcohol, they ate poorly (again, no detail is given), and in one of these two men, crypt cell megaloblastosis developed after four weeks of alcohol ingestion. Folacin replacement therapy reversed the intestinal mucosal changes, as well as the other evidences of folacin deficiency. Although this study has considerable interest in that the histological lesion of folacin deficiency in this small intestine is described, it appears that the authors do not consider that there is an interactive effect of ethanol and folacin deficiency in producing the intestinal lesion.

Four male chronic alcoholics between the ages of 39-59 years were studied by Halsted et al. (1973) with respect to the effects of ethanol and folate deficiency on intestinal absorption. The procedures followed in the four patients were similar in the first two patients (EC and GR), who received a regular hospital diet for three weeks (2200 Kcal) without alcohol, followed by a low folacin diet with alcohol at a level of 200 g/day; and then these patients were returned to the regular hospital diet, supplemented by folic acid (5 mg/day) for two weeks with alcohol at the previous dose. Another patient (ES) was given the regular hospital diet for a two week period, then a low folacin diet followed by the regular diet, supplemented by folic acid. Each of these latter diets was given for a period of two weeks. This patient did not receive alcohol during his hospital stay. The fourth patient was given the regular hospital diet throughout his hospital stay, with alcohol at the level of 300 g/day. Before folacin absorption studies were performed, he was additionally given alcohol at the level of 0.8 g/kg body weight by intrajejunal administration. After the study, he was maintained for two weeks without ethanol and restudied, with respect to intestinal resorption. Patients receiving the low-folacin diet, which was prepared by boiling foods, also received a vitamin and mineral supplement. Alcohol was given as 90-proof whiskey.

Induction of folacin deficiency was evaluated by hematologic parameters, by the FIGLU excretion test, by bone marrow examination, and by serum folacin values. Tests of intestinal absorption included the D-xylose test, estimation of fecal fat, and measurements of the jejunal absorption of tritiated folic acid (pteroylglutamic acid - ^{3}H-PGA). The absorption of the radiolabelled folate was determined by a triple lumen perfusion method. Trans-intestinal movements of fluid, sodium and glucose were also estimated. In the two patients who were given alcohol at a level of 200 gm/day with the low folate diet, reduction in serum folate levels was followed by decreased absorption of D-xylose, labelled folic acid, glucose, fluid and sodium. When these patients were returned to a regular hospital diet, supplemented by oral folic acid, but with continued alcohol administration, their intestinal absorption improved. Mild net secretion of fluid and sodium into the lumen of the intestine was noted in a patient who was abstinent on a low folacin diet and in the patient who took alcohol at a level of 300 g/day with a regular diet. In these patients examination of peroral intestinal biopsy specimens did not reveal any abnormalities of the jejunal mucosa. The authors conclude that combined dietary folacin deficiency and alcohol ingestion results in intestinal malabsorption, not only of folate per se, but also of other water-soluble substances. Folacin depletion as produced by the established protocol, did not induce malabsorption; nor did alcohol administration alone cause malabsorption as measured by these tests. It is suggested that impairment of nutritional status found in binge drinkers may be due to the combined effects of alcohol and limited dietary folacin intake.

Eichner et al. (1971) showed that, in alcoholics, diet-induced folacin deficiency develops more rapidly than in normal subjects. From these studies it seems clear that even if the combination of alcohol and a low-folacin diet contributes to intestinal malabsorption, whether or not overt folacin deficiency develops depends on pre-existing tissue folacin stores which may be depleted by prior ingestion of alcohol.

Thiamin malabsorption is induced by alcohol abuse. Tomasulo et al. (1968) studied the absorption of radiolabelled thiamin in 20 chronic alcoholic subjects (18 males and 2 females), and in ten non-alcoholic control subjects (5 males and 5 females). The average age in the two groups was similar. Alcoholic subjects were studied within seven days of admission to the hospital, after they had been drinking heavily. A very significant impairment in thiamin absorption was found in all the alcoholic subjects as compared with the non-alcoholic controls.

Further studies of thiamin absorption in alcoholics were performed by Thomson et al. (1970). Absorption of ^{35}S-thiamin hydrochloride was studied in 42 healthy subjects and 34 alcoholic subjects, of whom 17 had normal livers (according to the tests applied), 12 had fatty livers, and 5 had alcoholic cirrhosis. Thiamin malabsorption was found in the alcoholic patients who were malnourished and who also had fatty liver or cirrhosis. When these patients were given a 6-8 week period of nutritional rehabilitation on a high protein-vitamin supplemented diet, thiamin absorption returned to normal values. When alcohol was given either orally or parenterally to alcoholics without liver disease, four out of the 12 subjects showed reduced thiamin absorption. Adverse effects of ingested ethanol on thiamin absorption can presumably only be explained by assuming that the alcohol diffuses into the intestinal mucosa. This may possibly be the case, but since the observation was only made in one patient, it would seem appropriate to re-examine this finding. Of greater interest, perhaps, is the observation that the presence of ethanol in the gastrointestinal tract, as well as the chronic effects of alcohol on the intestine, can impair thiamin absorption.

Lindenbaum and Lieber (1975) have summarized scientific findings and opinions with respect to the interrelationship between alcoholism and intestinal malabsorption. They point out that, since it has been shown that certain types of nutritional deficiency can cause malabsorption, the relative effect of ethanol ingestion has been in question. They studied the effects of ethanol on certain specific intestinal functions on human subjects in a metabolic ward where the diet itself was adequate and was supplemented with vitamins. Of interest is the fact that the subjects who consisted in eight males, between the ages of 43-56, with a history of chronic alcoholism, were asymptomatic at the outset of the study, and their hematological status was within normal limits, as was liver function, serum folacin, serum vitamin B_{12} and both xylose and vitamin B_{12} absorption tests. While on study, four patients received a daily supplement of 200 μg of folic acid daily. Parenteral folic acid at a dose of 30 mg was given to certain subjects. The description of the diet suggests one with a high nutrient-calorie ratio. Vitamin B_{12} absorption was studied by the Schilling test, before, during and after administration of ethanol. Xylose absorption and fetal fat determinations were made at these same three periods. During the alcohol period, ethanol was substituted, iso-calorically, for carbohydrate in the diet, and, indeed, comprised 46-66% of total caloric intake (173-253 g/day). Findings were that vitamin B_{12} absorption was impaired in six out of the eight subjects. The vitamin B_{12} malabsorption was not corrected by giving intrinsic factor or pancreatin. Neither absorption of xylose nor fat was apparently inhibited by the administration of alcohol and, indeed, both serum and urinary xylose levels were increased during periods of ethanol ingestion. Perhaps this might be due to a delay in stomach emptying time, which is known to influence xylose apsorption. The fact that two subjects receiving the lowest dose of alcohol did not show vitamin B_{12} malabsorption, is taken by the authors to mean that perhaps this effect is dose-related.

We are still in doubt as to whether or not the effect of ethanol on the gastrointestinal tract, and more specifically, on the functions of the small intestine, is not rather to decrease ability of the intestinal mucosal cell to utilize nutrients and/or to transport nutrients. Based on the results of studies which have been cited, we can conclude that ethanol is a primary toxic agent with respect to the intestinal mucosal cell; that it does interfere with brush border function, and with the active transport of nutrients from the intestinal lumen into the mucosal cell; and that its toxic effects can impede carrier mediated transport of nutrients. Further, concomitant folacin deficiency, of dietary origin, which is common in alcoholics, can also produce intestinal malabsorption. Therefore, after review of current literature, it is apparent that, whereas studies in metabolic units of human subjects show clearcut evidence that ethanol alone is toxic to the intestine, in the real-life situation, malabsorption in alcoholics would tend to be multifactorial. It is not only multifactorial in the sense that it could be caused by associated pancreatic or hepatic disease, but also multifactorial in the sense that it is caused by the combined effects of ethanol and nutritional deficiency. A question which has still not been clarified is the extent to which malabsorption contributes to the vitamin malnutrition found in alcoholics.

SELECTED REFERENCES

Baraona, E., Pirola, R.C. and Lieber, C.S. 1974. Small intestinal damage and changes in cell population produced by ethanol ingestion in the rat. Gastroenterology 66: 226-234.

Barboriak, J.J. and Meade, R.C. 1969. Impairment of gastrointestinal processing of fat and protein by ethanol in rats. J. Nutr. 98: 373-378.

Dinoso, V.P., Chey, W.Y., Padow, D. et al. 1971. Gastrointestinal disorders in chronic alcoholics. Amer. J. Gastroenterol. 56: 209-215.

Editorial. 1977. Alcohol, gastritis and nutrient absorption. Nutr. Rev. 35: 8-10.

Eichner, E.R., Pierce, H.I. and Hillman, R.S. 1971. Folate balance in dietary-induced megaloblastic anemia. New Eng. J. Med. 284: 933-938.

Halsted, C.H., Robles, E.A. and Mezey, E. 1971. Decreased jejunal uptake of labelled folic acid (^{3}H-PGA) in alcoholic patients: Roles of alcohol and nutrition. New Eng. J. Med. 285: 701-706.

Halsted, C.H., Robles, E.A. and Mezey, E. 1973. Intestinal malabsorption in folate-deficient alcoholics. Gastroenterology 64: 526-532.

Hermos, J.A., Adams, W.H., Liu, Y.K., Sullivan, L.W. and Trier, J.S. 1972. Mucosa of the small intestine in folate-deficient alcoholics. Ann. Intern. Med. 76: 957-965.

Israel, Y., Salazar, I. and Rosenmann, E. 1968. Inhibitory effects of alcohol on intestinal amino acid transport in vivo and in vitro. J. Nutr. 96: 499-504.

Krasner, N., Carmichael, H.A., Russell, R.I., Thomson, D.G. and Cochran, K.M. 1976a. Alcohol and absorption from the small intestine. 2. Effects of ethanol on ATP and ATPase activities in guinea pig jejunum. Gut 17: 249-251.

Krasner, N., Cochran, K.M., Russell, R.I., Carmichael, H.A. and Thompson, G.G. 1976b. Alcohol absorption from the small intestine. 1. Impairment of absorption from the small intestine in alcoholics. Gut 17: 245-248.

Lindenbaum, J. and Lieber, C.S. 1975. Effects of chronic ethanol administration on intestinal absorption in man in the absence of nutritional deficiency. Ann. New York Acad. Sci. 252: 228-234.

Madzarovova-Nohejlova, J. 1971. Activite des disaccharidases intestinales chez l'adulte et chez le buveur chronique de biere de Pilsen. Biol. Gastroenterol. (Paris) 4: 325-332.

Malagelada, J-R., Owe, P. and Linsheer, W.G. 1974. Impaired absorption of micellar long-chain fatty acid in patients with alcoholic cirrhosis. Dig. Dis. 19: 1016.

Mezey, E. 1975. Intestinal function in chronic alcoholism. Ann. New York Acad. Sci. 252: 215-227.

Mezey, E., Jow, E., Slavin, R.E. and Tobon, F. 1970. Pancreatic function and intestinal absorption in chronic alcoholism. Gastroenterology 59: 657-664.

Perlow, W., Baraona, E. and Lieber, C.S. 1977. Symptomatic intestinal disaccharidase deficiency in alcoholics. Gastroenterology 72: 680-684.

Rubin, E., Ryback, B., Lindenbaum, J., Gerson, C.D., Walker, G. and Lieber, C.S. 1972. Ultrastructure changes in the small intestine induced by ethanol. Gastroenterology 53: 801-814.

Sardesai, E.M. and Orten, J.M. 1968. Effect of prolonged alcohol consumption in rats on pancreatic protein synthesis. J. Nutr. 96: 241-246.

Thomson, A.D., Baker, H. and Leevy, C.M. 1970. Patterns of ^{35}S-thiamin hydrochloride absorption in the malnourished alcoholic patient. J. Lab. Clin. Med. 76: 35-45.

Tomasulo, P.A., Kater, R.M.H. and Iber, F.L. 1968. Impairment of thiamin absorption in alcoholism. Amer. J. Clin. Nutr. 21: 1340-1344.

Adverse Effects of Alcohol on Nutritional Status

Adverse effects of alcohol on nutritional status may be apparent or real. It is recognized that following infusion or ingestion of alcohol, nutrient disposition is altered. This may result in the transient reduction of blood levels of nutrients or an increase in the urinary excretion. Acute nutritional effects of this type are rapidly reversed when ethanol intake is discontinued. On the other hand, chronic alcoholics are likely to develop malnutrition of multifactorial origin. Malnutrition in the alcoholic may simultaneously or progressively affect more than one nutrient, and the evolution of these nutritional deficiencies shows that the production of each new deficiency may, in one way or another, be dependent on the deficiencies that have previously existed. Although diminished nutrient intake is a common etiologic factor, accounting for much of the nutritional disease in alcoholics, low nutrient intake can no longer be considered as an explanation for all the various nutritional syndromes as seen in association with chronic alcoholism.

Nutritional deficiencies in alcoholics can be classified by cause, effect, sequence and interrelationships.

GENERAL CAUSES OF MALNUTRITION IN ALCOHOLISM

Two general statements can be made: that certain classes of alcoholics, particularly those in indigent and "skid-row" categories, have frequently been shown to have inadequate nutrient intakes, particularly of the water-soluble vitamins; and also, alcohol itself interferes with nutrient utilization. Interactions of alcohol toxicity and malnutrition lead to deficiency syndromes which differ in clinical, hematological, and biochemical characteristics from nutrient deficiencies caused by diet alone. Confusion, which has arisen in medical and scientific literature, with respect to the interpretation of blood levels of nutrients in alcoholics, stems from two causes. In the first place, it has not been adequately appreciated that, if a nutrient cannot be utilized, then its level in the blood may be elevated rather than depressed. Secondly, insufficient recognition has been given to the timing of studies of alcoholic patients. Since the adverse effects of alcohol on nutrition and, more particularly, on nutrient levels may be acute and rapidly reversible, it is clear that if studies are delayed after the withdrawal of alcohol, it may not be possible to compare the nutritional status of alcoholic patients during enforced abstinence with those when the patient is actively consuming alcohol.

Discussion of effects of alcohol on the utilization of individual nutrients is often inappropriate, since deficiency of one nutrient or impaired metabolism of one nutrient may affect utilization of others. It is more realistic to discuss nutritional diseases of alcoholics under a broad diagnostic classification to include anemias, neuropathies, hepatic and cutaneous disease.

NUTRITIONAL ANEMIAS AND ALCOHOLISM

Alcohol abuse has been associated with the development of hematologic abnormalities. These abnormalities may be due to direct toxic effects of ethanol, nutritional deficits, or anemias caused by additive or synergistic effects of ethanol toxicity and nutrient deficiency. Hematologic defects in alcoholics include vacuolation of precursor cells of the erythroid (red blood cell) and myeloid (white blood cell) series, macrocytosis without folate deficiency, megaloblastic erythropoiesis, and anemia secondary to folate deficiency, sideroblastic anemia with evidence of abnormal metabolism of vitamin B6, sideroblastic anemia without identification of the vitamin B6 defect, iron deficiency after hemorrhage into the GI tract, chronic hemolytic anemia with cirrhosis, transient hemolysis with hyperlipemia, thrombocytopenia, granulocytopenia, and depressed leukocyte motilization. This itemized list of hematologic abnormalities associated with alcoholism is modified from that developed by Eichner and Hillman (1971).

A direct toxic effect of ethanol on hemopoiesis was first suggested by Jandl (1955). Lindenbaum and Lieber (1969) demonstrated that when alcohol is given to alcoholics during a period of abstinence when they are maintained on an adequate diet with vitamin supplements, abnormalities of hemopoiesis develop. These abnormalities include 1) vacuolation of bone marrow pronormoblasts; 2) vacuolation of pro-myelocytes which is less consistent and only occurs with larger doses of alcohol; and 3) normalization of red and white cell precursor mor-phology after withdrawal of the alcohol. The vacuolation of the red and white cell precursors, during the period of alcohol administration, appeared to be dose-related. During the time of alcohol intake, there was a variable reduction in the platelet count. The authors comment that vacuolation of red cell precursors has also been observed in riboflavin-deficient baboons (Kondi and Foy, 1964), in phenylalanine-deficient children (Sherman et al., 1964), and in patients treated with large doses of chloramphenicol (Rosenbach et al., 1960). Whereas the authors intimate that the possibility exists that the observed vac-uolation of the bone marrow precursor cells could be due to inadequate utilization of flavin compounds, or inhibition of protein synthesis, they also note that during the period of ethanol administration, when the vacuolation developed, the patients were receiving a high riboflavin supplement, as well as a diet rich in protein.

Hines and Cowan (1970) investigated the effects of alcohol ad-ministration on abstinent alcoholics with respect to several indices of hemopoiesis. In their three subjects, hematocrit values were reduced to anemic levels during the period of alcohol administration. Serum iron was elevated and plasma iron turnover markedly increased. Decreased red cell iron utilization was demonstrated. In the bone marrow, both megaloblastic and sideroblastic changes were found. Ring sideroblasts were identified in the bone marrow of two of the subjects. The serum levels of folate and pyridoxal phosphate were measured sequentially during the thirty day period of alcohol administration. In all three subjects, serum levels of both of these nutrients were progressively reduced by the alcohol (as whiskey). The reduction in serum pyridoxal phosphate levels to some extent paralleled the degree of sideroblastosis. Intravenous administration of pyridoxine caused an increase in serum pyridoxal phosphate levels, but these levels did not reach pre-alcohol levels until nine weeks after alcohol withdrawal. Administration of pyridoxal phosphate was followed by reticulocytosis, and disappear-ance of ring sideroblasts from the bone marrow. Administration of pharmacologic doses of folic acid (pteroylmonoglutamic acid) was followed by lessening in the degree of megaloblastosis, but meg-aloblastic changes in the bone marrow persisted.

The direct toxic effect of alcohol on erythropoiesis has been further studied by Hourihan and Weir (1970). They studied alcoholic patients newly admitted to a private psychiatric hospital in Dublin. Bone marrow studies of 23 such patients were carried out within two hours of hospitalization and again, 2-7 days later. Vacuolation of hemopoietic cell precursors and sideroblastosis were found in the initial bone marrow specimens, but these changes disappeared after periods of abstinence. Following admission, serum iron levels which had been initially high dropped progressively. None of these patients were considered to be undernourished by the authors. The authors used the term "dyshemopoiesis" to describe the observed morphological changes in the bone marrow. They believe that their findings are consistent with defective hemoglobin synthesis as well as toxic ethanolic effects upon cell structure within the bone marrow.

Macrocytosis of the peripheral blood erythrocytes is perhaps the most consistent finding in actively drinking alcoholics. In the author's experience of community and clinic nutrition surveys and research, the finding of a mean corpuscular volume above 92 cubic micron in association with a low or deficient level of plasma folacin is indicative of alcohol abuse. Among episodic drinkers, these findings are not necessarily indicative of nutritional folacin deficiency, since erythrocyte folacin levels may be within normal limits and megaloblastic anemia is absent. Herbert et al. (1963) reviewed the fact that Bianco and Jolliffe had noted the macrocytosis of alcoholics in 1938; they then commented: "In view of these findings, we are inclined to regard the macrocytosis of the alcohol addict not as a manifestation of inability on the part of the liver to store a hematopoietic principle, but as an extrinsic deficiency of some necessary hematopoietic substance required to maintain normocytosis."

In a group of 70 patients with alcoholism and varying degrees of hepatic dysfunction, Herbert et al. (1963) found that only 7% had normal serum folate concentrations. Macro-ovalocytes were present in the peripheral blood smears of all of these patients who had serum folate concentrations below 3 ng/ml.

Macrocytosis, unassociated with folate deficiency, has also been documented by Chanarin (1969). There is indeed evidence that the macrocytosis of alcoholics unattended by definitive folate deficiency may be a manifestation of the toxic effect of ethanol analogous to the vacuolation of precursor cells in the bone marrow.

Wu et al. (1974) studied 63 patients who, on a chronic basis, had been consuming more than 80 gm ethanol daily. Macrocytosis was present in 89% of the subjects, but in only a few was this associated with anemia. Megaloblastic changes were found in about one-third of the bone marrow samples. Decreases in the serum, erythrocyte and liver folate levels were found in approximately one-third of the patients. Macrocytosis was reversed when alcohol was withdrawn, but persisted when the subjects were given folate supplements if alcohol intake was not also discontinued. The authors comment that: "Macrocytosis is one of the commonest abnormalities in alcoholics in the U.K." They also believe that this is due to the direct action of alcohol on developing red cells and that it is not necessarily due to folate deficiency.

Doubt can no longer exist that ethanol has a primary toxic effect on the developing hemopoietic cells in the bone marrow, and further that damage to these cells by the toxic agent impairs their capacity to utilize nutrients required for cell maturation. Alcohol abuse leads to impairments in the structure and function of the cells of the hemopoietic system. The question which must be answered is whether we can explain the functional defects in terms of impaired nutrient utilization.

The demonstration by many investigators that sideroblasts are commonly present in the bone marrows of alcoholic patients gave rise to the question of why iron should be deposited in these cells and not utilized for heme synthesis. Hillman (1975) has described mitochondrial damage within red cell precursors and, indeed, this is a common toxic effect of alcohol on the cell structure. Abnormal mitochondria in alcoholic marrows have been demonstrated by electron microscopy.

It is proposed that hemopoietic function, confined to the mitochondria, would be diminished under the circumstance of alcohol damage. These functions would include two major steps in heme synthesis: condensation of glycine and succinyl Co-A to form delta-aminolevulinic acid and the incorporation of iron into protoporphyrin—the terminal step in heme formation.

Alcohol blocks the interconversion of vitamers of vitamin B_6. Alcoholics exhibit defects of hemopoietic function, indicating malfunctioning and/or absolute deficiency of vitamin B_6. Hillman (1975) has suggested that the accumulation of iron in alcoholic red cell precursors is not only due to defects in heme synthesis, but perhaps also to the prolongation of the intermitotic time which could increase the absorption of iron into the developing red cell. It is suggested by this author that the characteristic development of sideroblasts is therefore associated with the megaloblastic state.

Abnormalities of vitamin B_6 metabolism have been identified in alcoholics. Hines (1975) showed that in alcoholic subjects without evidence of liver disease, serum pyridoxal phosphate levels are decreased. This same investigator determined the effect of alcohol on the conversion of pyridoxine to pyridoxal phosphate in four chronic alcoholic subjects before and after administration of alcohol. Prior to alcohol administration, that is, during a period of abstinence, erythrocyte hemolysate pyridoxal kinase activities of alcoholic volunteers were not significantly different from those of age-matched control non-alcoholic subjects. However, after alcohol ingestion there was a reduction in pyridoxal kinase activity. Preliminary studies have been carried out in an attempt to identify an inhibitory factor of the pyridoxal kinase system in alcoholics who are actively drinking. On the basis of a rather small body of data, it is postulated that in some alcoholic subjects, who are well nourished, a protein-bound plasma inhibitor of pyridoxal kinase is generated during the time of excessive alcohol ingestion.

Lumeng and Li (1974) also studied plasma pyridoxal phosphate levels in alcoholic subjects. They selected 66 alcoholics who had normal liver function tests and hematologic findings. Thirty-five of these had plasma pyridoxal phosphate concentrations, less than 5 ng/ml, which was the lowest value encountered in their 94 control subjects. This was accepted as evidence of abnormal pyridoxal phosphate metabolism in the alcoholics. The low plasma pyridoxal phosphate levels in the alcoholics were not associated with decreased pyridoxal kinase or pyridoxine phosphate oxidase activities in the intact erythrocytes of these people. They further found that acetaldehyde rather than ethanol impaired the formation of pyridoxal phosphate from pyridoxal, pyridoxine, and pyridoxine phosphate by erythrocytes. Using broken cell preparations of erythrocytes, it was found that the effect of acetaldehyde was mediated by the B_6-phosphate phosphatase, causing an accelerated breakdown of phosphorylated B_6 vitamers in erythrocytes.

Apparent differences in findings of Hines and Lumeng and Li with respect to the derangement of vitamin B_6 metabolism in the erythrocytes of alcoholics may be explained by variation in methodology. Presently, however, while it is accepted that there is a defect in the utilization of vitamin B_6 in the erythrocytes of alcohol abusers and a consequent interference with iron utilization for heme synthesis, the precise nature of the metabolic defect has not been well defined.

Erythrocyte conversion of pyridoxine to pyridoxal phosphate has been shown to be increased by administration of riboflavin (Anderson et al., 1976). Riboflavin deficiency is recognized as a common complication of chronic alcoholism (Rosenthal et al., 1973). Question may be asked whether riboflavin deficiency contributes to, or may partially explain, the defect in vitamin B_6 metabolism within erythrocytes in alcoholics. Riboflavin is required for the conversion of pyridoxine phosphate to pyridoxal phosphate (Goldsmith, 1975; Wada and Snell, 1961).

It was demonstrated by Eichner et al. (1971) that in alcoholic subjects megaloblastic hemopoiesis develops rapidly when ethanol ingestion is combined with a folacin deficient diet. These authors make three inferences from their studies of two alcoholic volunteers. The studies of these two men strongly suggest an inverse relationship between folacin stores and the rate of development of folate deficiency on a folacin deficient diet with alcohol administration. They further declare that ethanol appears to accelerate megaloblastic changes.

These investigators observed an association between ethanol ingestion and the development of megaloblastosis, folacin deficiency, and elevation in serum iron levels. Conversely, they found that a reduction in serum iron levels and normalization of the hematologic picture followed parenteral administration of folic acid (pteroylmonoglutamic acid). It is suggested that the initial factor in the ineffective hemopoiesis induced by ethanol is folacin deficiency, or an inability to utilize folacin (Eichner et al., 1971).

Some very interesting comments have been made by this same group of investigators, pertinent to relationships between ethanol ingestion, folacin status and anemia in alcoholics. Eichner et al. (1972), in a study of skid-row and middle to upper-class alcoholics, found variability in the incidence and type of anemia in the group. In the skid-row alcoholics, iron deficiency anemia was common and this is partially explained by the fact that people in this group were in the habit of giving blood through a commercial blood bank operation at frequent intervals. A relationship is further pointed out between folacin and iron status. Summarizing their own findings as well as those of other authors, the investigators comment:

> "Patients (alcoholics) with ineffective erythropoiesis often have increased levels of serum iron and increased marrow iron stores because of continued recycling iron from short-lived red cells. When these patients are treated with folic acid, the serum iron rapidly declines and abnormal sideroblasts disappear as normal erythropoiesis is restored ... Marrow iron stores may also decrease during the first 1-2 weeks after normal erythropoiesis is restored ... A decline in marrow iron stores is to be expected during the response to folic acid as iron becomes incorporated into the newly formed red cells ... Some patients with megaloblastic anemia may become iron deficient during response to folic acid."

While it is reasonable to accept the premise that folacin deficiency does influence the utilization of other nutrients by the red cell or red cell precursor, it is premature to assume that folacin deficiency is more important than a metabolic defect in the utilization of vitamin B_6 in this regard.

Complicating the issue of the folacin status of alcoholics is the observed decline in the plasma folacin levels of alcohol abusers independent of other evidence of folacin deficiency. Ethanol ingestion or infusion causes a fall in plasma folate levels, but apparently not as a result of depletion of folacin stores. *In vitro* experiments have shown that this is not an assay artifact. Eichner and Hillman (1973), who made these observations, further suggested that perhaps alcohol interferes with the delivery of N^5-methyltetrahydrofolic acid from storage areas.

A partial block in the rate of release of tissue folacin stores has been proposed as a possible mechanism leading to the speedy depression in plasma methyltetrahydrofolate levels, as well as early induction of megaloblastic erythropoiesis following ethanol ingestion. Lane *et al.* (1976), who made these associations based on experimental data, obtained no evidence that alcohol ingestion increases the urinary loss of the vitamin or its catabolic product.

TABLE 8.1 ADVERSE EFFECTS OF ETHANOL ON HEMOPOIESIS WITH SEQUENTIAL DEFECTS IN NUTRIENT UTILIZATION.

Hemopoietic Defect	Mechanism
1. Vacuolization of red and white cell precursors Macrocytosis	Toxic effect of ethanol
2. Megaloblastosis	Impaired folacin availability or utilization
3. Sideroblastosis	Mitochondrial dysfunction Defect in vitamin B_6 utilization

NUTRITIONAL FACTORS IN THE DEVELOPMENT OF ORGANIC BRAIN SYNDROMES AND NEUROPATHIES IN ALCOHOLICS

The neuropsychiatric disorders and syndromes which have been associated with alcoholism are numerous. Feuerlein (1976) includes alcohol withdrawal syndrome, delirium tremens, alcoholic hallucinosis, Wernicke-Korsakoff syndrome, seizures, tremor, Marchiafava-Bignami disease, and central pontine myelinolysis, alcoholic amblyopia, alcoholic cerebellar degeneration, cerebral atrophy, alterations of personality and chronic polyneuropathy. Several of these disorders have a nutritional etiology, including the Wernicke-Korsakoff syndrome, with associated polyneuropathy, the Marchiafava-Bignami disease which may be associated with the Wernicke-Korsakoff syndrome, and possibly alcoholic amblyopia. Whereas in the case of the Wernicke-Korsakoff syndrome and polyneuropathy associated with beri-beri, there is strong evidence of thiamin deficiency as a causal factor, the specific nutritional disorder underlying other alcoholic neurological conditions has not been defined.

As with other alcoholic diseases, the neuropathies and encephalopathies seen in alcoholics are either entirely due to the toxic effects of ethanol or to an interaction of nutritional deficiency with alcohol toxicity. Current opinion upholds the concept that the Wernicke-Korsakoff syndrome, possibly the Marchiafava-Bignami disease and alcoholic polyneuropathy are clinical manifestations of a thiamin dependency syndrome. Since the alcoholic frequently has multiple nutritional deficiencies due to inadequate nutrient intake, malabsorption, or inadequate nutrient utilization, it is not surprising that the alcoholic with brain or neural disorders displays signs and symptoms indicative of the coexistence of several deficiency states including thiamin, riboflavin, pyridoxine, and niacin deficiency (Table 8.2). However, reversability or prevention of specific neuropsychiatric alcoholic disorders such as the Wernicke-Korsakoff syndrome, require the administration of a specific vitamin, namely thiamin, as well as alcohol withdrawal.

TABLE 8.2 NEUROLOGICAL DISORDERS ASSOCIATED WITH PRIMARY OR CONDITIONED NUTRITIONAL DEFICIENCY IN ALCOHOLICS.

Clinical Disorder	Nutritional Deficiency
Wernicke-Korsakoff syndrome	Thiamin
Peripheral neuropathy	Thiamin Vitamin B_6
Pellagrous psychosis	Niacin

From the historic standpoint, our knowledge of the Wernicke-Korsakoff syndrome describes the evolution of knowledge of the effects of chronic alcohol abuse, on cellular function in general, and on neural tissues in particular. The Wernicke syndrome per se consists in an acute confusional state accompanied by ocular abnormalities including nystagmus, paralyses of the ocular muscles including the lateral rectus, weakness of conjugate gaze, ataxia, or loss of balance, and commonly, a polyneuropathy with weakness of the legs as a presenting symptom. This symptomatology may be accompanied by mild fever, tachycardia, and/or evidence of liver disease. There is a variable depression of the state of consciousness, commonly with stupor from which the patient can be aroused. The disease occurs in certain chronic alcoholics who have abstained from food or who have eaten irregularly for long periods of time.

Wernicke's syndrome may occur occasionally in patients without a history of alcohol abuse, who suffer either from gross malabsorption syndromes, metastatic malignancies, or who have been receiving prolonged intravenous therapy without hyperalimentation. Untreated Wernicke's syndrome commonly progresses into Korsakoff's psychosis, characterized by a gross memory deficit and confabulation. Wernicke's syndrome is well described by Riggs and Boles (1944-45). These authors consider that Wernicke's syndrome is a form of thiamin deficiency to be found in alcoholics. They further intimate that in those cases where a history of alcoholism cannot be obtained, it nevertheless may exist. They point out the fact that it was Jolliffe *et al.* (1941) who first offered the suggestion that this disease is an expression of "a nutritional deficiency state, and that alcohol is implicated only by reason of its effects upon nutrition." Earlier workers had described brain lesions occurring in experimental animals as a result of thiamin deficiency. Their findings had influenced the belief that Wernicke's syndrome was also a thiamin deficiency disease (Zimmerman, 1939; Alexander, 1940; Evans *et al.*, 1942).

Cases described by Riggs and Boles (1944-45) showed evidence of multiple nutritional deficiencies including emaciation, peripheral edema, stomatitis, and cheilosis. A common complication of Wernicke's syndrome or encephalopathy is profound hypothermia. Hunter (1976), describing a case of Wernicke's syndrome complicated by hypothermia, notes that this sign may mask other symptoms and delay diagnosis. It is suggested by this author that in any alcoholic presenting with severe hypothermia, thiamin should be administered. This therapeutic advice is a direct extension of the viewpoint that the syndrome is reversible by administration of therapeutic doses of thiamin.

The most complete description and discussion of the Wernicke-Korsakoff syndrome has been given by Victor *et al.* (1971). These authors made a strong plea for the unity of the Wernicke-Korsakoff syndrome, pointing out that, whereas usually there is a progression of symptoms and signs from the acute Wernicke's syndrome (encephalopathy) to Korsakoff's psychosis, the signs of Wernicke's encephalopathy may coexist with Korsakoff's psychosis. In their description of brain pathology found at autopsy, they describe focal necrosis of brain cells within the midbrain, thalamus and pons, with symmetrical loss of brain cells and myelin degeneration within nuclei in these areas of the brain, and more particularly, in relation to the ventricles. In some cases which came to autopsy, patients had died when Korsakoff's psychosis was present, but causes of death included other alcoholic diseases and/or intercurrent infection.

In the monograph by Victor *et al.* (1971), the authors subscribe to the viewpoint that the Wernicke-Korsakoff syndrome is a thiamin deficiency disease, but that the acute phase (Wernicke's syndrome) responds better to administration of thiamin than does the chronic phase of the disease (Korsakoff's psychosis). They further present the hypothesis that the Wernicke-Korsakoff syndrome is a pure form of thiamin deficiency, while endemic beri-beri of the "dry type" may be a multiple vitamin deficiency involving several B vitamins. We are reminded of the work of Rinehart *et al.* (1949), who produced thiamin deficiency in the rhesus monkey. In this species, central nervous system lesions were similar in some respects to those of the Wernicke-Korsakoff syndrome.

Victor *et al.* (1971) further shows that several alcoholic diseases of the central nervous system should be considered under the umbrella diagnosis of the Wernicke-Korsakoff syndrome. These include the Marchiafava-Bignami disease, clinically manifested by dissociative function of the cerebral hemispheres and pathologically by a symmetrical degeneration of the central portion of the corpus callosum. If, in fact, we are to accept the idea that the Marchiafava-Bignami syndrome is a special form of alcoholic thiamin deficiency, only to be distinguished from the Wernicke-Korsakoff syndrome by the peculiar distribution of cerebral lesions, then it should be possible to find biochemical indices of thiamin deficiency in such patients, as well as responsiveness to thiamin administration. In three cases of the Marchiafava-Bignami disease, described by Lhermitte *et al.* (1977), biochemical evidence of thiamin deficiency was not obtained, nor is the effect of thiamin administration mentioned.

Another alcoholic disease of the central nervous system, alcoholic cerebellar degeneration, is also accepted by Victor *et al.* (1971) as an extension of Wernicke's disease; a suggestion which would have general acceptability. Elevated blood pyruvate levels have been found by Platt and Lu (1939) in cases of endemic beriberi. Similarly, fasting blood pyruvate levels in untreated patients with Wernicke's disease may be elevated as demonstrated by Victor *et al.* (1957). A non-specificity of blood pyruvate levels in the measure of thiamin deficiency has been noted and therefore, the erythrocyte transketolase activity, a functional test of thiamin status, has been measured in patients with Wernicke's disease. Prior to treatment with thiamin, there is marked reduction in transketolase activity with a reversal to normal soon after the administration of thiamin (Victor *et al.*, 1971).

The question has been asked why alcoholics should develop signs and symptoms of a pure thiamin deficiency. Whereas inadequate intake in relation to requirements is a possible explanation, the diet of the alcoholic developing the Wernicke-Korsakoff syndrome tends to be deficient in all nutrients rather than being a specifically thiamin deficient diet. It was noted by Victor *et al.* (1971) and by others, that among patients with the Wernicke-Korsakoff syndrome, most, including both men and women, are chronic alcoholics and not binge drinkers, and may therefore be able to return to an adequate food intake between episodes of drinking.

Thiamin malabsorption has been demonstrated by several groups of workers in actively drinking alcoholics (Tomasulo *et al.*, 1968; Thomson *et al.*, 1970). There is an increasing body of evidence to suggest that such syndromes as the Wernicke-Korsakoff syndrome do not develop because of a simple thiamin deficiency associated with decreased intake or malabsorption, but that cells and fibers within the ethanol damaged brain and peripheral nervous system are thiamin dependent. Beriberi or classical thiamin deficiency varies in its manifestations, and includes a dry polyneuritic form and wet beriberi, characterized by edema and cardiac abnormalities. Phosphorylation of thiamin to form the active coenzyme, thiamin pyrophosphate, is inhibited in the ethanol damaged liver. Patients with Korsakoff's psychosis have been shown to have low values of thiamin pyrophosphate in the blood (Sinclair, 1972).

A polio encephalomalacia has been found in dogs, cats, and foxes in association with chronic thiamin deficiency (Reed *et al.*, 1977; Jubb *et al.*, 1956; Evans *et al.*, 1942). Signs of the encephalopathy described in dogs by Reed *et al.* (1977) responded to administration of pharmacological doses of thiamin hydrochloride (250 mg, given parenterally). Two distinctive abnormalities in thiamin metabolism occur in chronic alcoholics: a phosphorylating defect of thiamin and an apotransketolase deficiency (Sauberlich, 1967). In one of the thiamin-responsive inborn errors of metabolism, the subacute necrotizing encephalomyelopathy, there is a lack of thiamin triphosphate in the neural tissue of the brain (Pincus *et al.*, 1973). Patients may respond to pharmacologic doses of thiamin. Whether alcoholic brain toxicity can cause an abnormality similar to this inborn defect is unclear, but there is evidence to support the theory that thiamin may have a specific role in neurophysiology which is independent of its coenzyme function: that is, in maintaining the integrity of the neuron (Itokawa and Cooper, 1970; Tanphaichitr, 1976).

GENETIC DETERMINATION OF FOOD AND NUTRIENT REQUIREMENTS OF ALCOHOLICS

Recent studies have indicated that replacement of food intake by alcohol intake may have different consequences for different individuals, and these differences have a genetic basis. Blass and Gibson (1977) reported on the existence of abnormalities of a thiamin-dependent enzyme in patients with the Wernicke-Korsakoff syndrome. On culturing fibroblasts from patients with this syndrome and from control lines, they found that the transketolase enzyme in the fibroblasts from the patients bound thiamin pyrophosphate less strongly than in the controls. The data suggest abnormalities in the transketolase enzyme of these individuals, which may be due to a structural mutation. It is proposed that these patients, because of a genetic defect, are vulnerable to develop thiamin deficiency with neurological manifestations. If their thiamin intake is below their requirements, it is suggested that decreased activity of the transketolase enzyme is an essential abnormality of the Wernicke-Korsakoff syndrome.

The Wernicke-Korsakoff syndrome has been found to occur more frequently among Europeans than non-Europeans on thiamin-deficient diets, and perhaps this can be interpreted as further supportive evidence for a genetic determination of this neurological complication of alcoholism (Van Itallie et al., 1974). The broader question now has to be decided as to whether eating habits of alcoholics and particularly their consumption of specific nutrients, may have different consequences for different people showing biochemical individuality.

ALCOHOLIC HEART DISEASE

Primary alcoholic heart disease has been variously identified and classified such that each author or group of authors suggest their own theories of etiology. McDonald et al. (1971) reply on three diagnostic criteria:

1. Appearance of signs and symptoms of cardiomyopathy (disease of the heart muscle), plus persistant cardiomegaly (enlargement of the heart).
2. History of alcohol abuse.
3. Inability to find any other cause for the heart disease except heavy alcohol intake.

Brigden and Robinson (1964) include under alcoholic heart disease "isolated non-coronary myocardial disease." These authors reported on

50 patients seen at two London hospitals between 1952 and 1963; the criteria for their inclusion in the series being a prolonged history of high consumption of alcohol and evidence of heart disease which was not due to hypertension, coronary artery disease, valvular disease or any other disorder known to cause heart disease. Included by these authors as having alcoholic heart disease are those with wet beriberi, arrhythmias and chronic myocardial failure. It is of interest that three of their patients who had beriberi heart failure were heavy beer drinkers, and had had a previous partial gastrectomy. It is suggested that the partial gastrectomy could have contributed to the thiamin deficiency. Among their patients who did not show the signs of beriberi, there was a small group with severe heart failure and evidence of very low cardiac output and another group with recurrent heart failure, sometimes associated with atrial fibrillation. Common findings on autopsy examination of the non-beriberi cases were hypertrophy of the left ventricle, dilation of the right ventricle, and both atria, and some areas of cardiac muscle degeneration, sometimes with patchy fibrosis. In the cases of cardiac beriberi, satisfactory therapeutic response occurred when thiamin was given and alcohol withdrawn. In some of the other patients, amelioration in the cardiac condition was associated with total abstinence.

Douglas Talbott (1975) describes three entities under the general heading of primary alcoholic heart disease: 1) nutritional type; 2) toxic type; and 3) conductive type. This author also discusses secondary alcoholic heart disease in which an excessive consumption of alcohol imposes an adverse effect on a heart affected by prior pathology; for example, the finding that ingestion of large amounts of alcohol can cause sudden death by cardiac arrest. The nutritional type of primary alcoholic heart disease is considered to be synonymous with wet beriberi. Among a series of 1500 alcoholics, the author only found 10% with the nutritional type of alcoholic heart disease, and this relatively low incidence is considered to be due to intake by alcoholic patients of breads and other cereals fortified with thiamin. The toxic type accounted for 80% of the patients in this series.

It is considered that cardiac changes result from the direct toxic effects of ethanol on the myocardium. Cardiac toxicity of ethanol causes fragmentation and destruction of the cardiac muscle fibers, loss of contractile elements, presence of swollen mitochondria, and intercellular edema fluid, accumulation of glycogen, and altered permeability of the muscle cell membrane. Lipid deposition is also increased. Focal areas of inflammatory cell response may be found and also replacement of cardiac muscle by scar tissue. The suggestion is made that a diagnosis of the toxic form of primary alcoholic heart disease may be made if the following combination of physical signs exists or coexists: an enlarged liver, skin changes suggestive of alcohol abuse including spider angiomata, red palms, and rhinophyma (large red nose), internal hemorrhoids and radiologically demonstrable esophageal varices. Additionally, diagnosis requires a history of "reasonable nutritional intake prior to presentation and a failure of thiamin to alleviate the cardiac clinical abnormalities." There should also be an absence of any arrhythmias. Recommended treatment includes absolute abstinence, prolonged bedrest, routine therapy for heart failure, and a high protein diet. In the conductive form of primary alcoholic heart disease, theory is advanced that conduction abnormalities result from electrolyte imbalance. Prevention or control of arrhythmias by this investigator has been through administration of magnesium and potassium in a fructose base, given by the oral route.

Causes and effects of magnesium deficiency in alcoholics are described by Flink (1971). Low intakes of magnesium, coupled with increased excretion, contribute to the magnesium deficit. Evidence is given that the cardiac pathology found in alcoholic heart disease is similar to that of magnesium deficiency induced in rats. It was also pointed out that magnesium deficiency may potentiate effects of thiamin deficit. Hypokalemia, which is common in alcoholics, can cause the arrhythmias associated with the conductive form of primary alcoholic heart disease. Hypokalemia occurs not only with acute alcohol withdrawal, but also may occur while alcoholics are still imbibing ethanol (Vetter et al., 1967).

The natural course of alcoholic cardiomyopathy, apparently the toxic type, has been discussed by Demakis et al. (1975). These investigators studied 57 patients with alcoholic cardiomyopathy and followed them up for an average time of 40.5 months. Among their patients, in 15 the clinical status improved (group A); in 12 the status became stable (group B); and in 30 there was a deterioration (group C). Within group A, 73% of patients abstained from alcohol; in group B, 25% abstained, and in group C, only 13% abstained. In the C group, 24 patients died in an average time of 36 months.

As indicated by this report, there is strong evidence suggesting that ethanol itself is toxic to the heart, and that a toxic effect of ethanol may be reversible. Schwartz et al. (1975) described a chronic alcoholic with congestive cardiomyopathy. He had been a heavy consumer of whiskey for about twenty years, drinking about 16 oz. of whiskey/day. Although initial angiographic and hemodynamic evidence of left ventricular dysfunction was present, this was completely reversed after one year of abstinence. At an 18 month follow-up he was also asymptomatic, and required no cardiac medications. This amelioration of his cardiac condition was apparently maintained despite the fact that he was drinking moderately (2-4 oz. of whiskey/week) from 13 months after the initial episode. A contributory factor in the good outcome may well have been the fact that, whereas initially he had been a heavy cigarette smoker, he stopped smoking after he came under observation. No detail is given by the authors concerning his diet, but his food intake and nutrition were said to be "good."

The pathophysiology of primary alcoholic heart disease is still not fully explained. Bing *et al.* (1975) emphasized that ethanol can cause changes in cardiac contractility and metabolism. However, manifestation of these disorders induced by alcohol on the heart by demonstrable functional change requires prolonged consumption of excess of alcohol. Whereas the inherent property of contractility of muscle, including heart muscle, lies in the protein actomyosin, which contracts under the influence of ATP, the particulate fraction of muscle known as the sarcoplasmic reticulum contains the relaxing factor. The sarcoplasmic reticulum (or rather the relaxing granules within the system) induce relaxation by inducing the movement of calcium ions such that Ca^{++} are pumped out of the membrane of the sarcoplasmic reticulum granules and allowed to combine with the contractile elements of the muscle. This course of events occurs during contraction, and during relaxation the Ca^{++} return to the sarcoplasmic reticulum granules. The mitochondria may also have the function of storing calcium ions and, as such, may contribute to the function of relaxation of contractile elements (myofibrils). Mitochondria are also, of course, the prime site for production of ATP. In dogs, it has been found that prolonged alcohol administration causes abnormalities in calcium uptake and binding by both the sarcoplasmic reticulum and the mitochondria. This may lead to an impairment in the relaxation of the contractile elements of the heart.

Rubin *et al.* (1976) investigated the effects of chronic alcohol consumption on skeletal muscle in baboons, in an alcoholic patient, and in a group of volunteers who were induced to consume alcohol. Heavy microsomal fraction isolates from muscle biopsies showed diminished calcium uptake. Membranes of sarcoplasmic reticulum also exhibited decreased calcium uptake in several of the human volunteers. It was considered by the investigators not to be due to the presence of alcohol in the tissues, since studies were conducted after intake of alcohol was discontinued. Ultrastructure changes in muscle were induced by alcohol administration in the baboons employed in this study, as well as in the human volunteers, despite the fact that the latter were provided with a high energy-high nutrient diet with multivitamin and mineral supplements. Investigators imply that this study gives additional evidence for the direct toxic action of alcohol on muscle tissue, and by extrapolation on heart muscle tissue.

The dogma that in primary alcoholic heart disease of the non-beriberi type, cardiac damage is entirely due to the ethanol, and is not a nutritional problem, can be argued if the definition of nutrition includes the utilization of nutrients, e.g. calcium, by the cell.

The observation that beer drinking has been more commonly associated with the development of primary alcoholic heart disease than consumption of other alcoholic beverages in the United States was discussed by Alexander (1966). Whereas this author considered it desirable to investigate the effects of specific ingredients of beer on the heart with respect to toxic action, it is questionable whether such research is necessary in view of the fact that ethanol per se has been shown to produce the characteristic cardiac changes. It should, however, be remembered that cobalt intoxication due to addition of cobalt to beers has been incriminated as a cause of cardiotoxicity. In 1957, cobalt was first added to beer in order to enhance the foam-keeping properties. In the following ten years, several series of cases of cobalt-induced cardiomyopathy were reported. The disease could be differentiated from primary alcoholic heart disease by the presence of pericardial effusion, and usually the presence of polycythemia. Sullivan et al. (1968) determined the cobalt concentrations in the hearts of patients who died of heart disease after drinking cobalt-containing beers in the Omaha, Nebraska region. Cobalt concentrations were significantly greater in the hearts of these patients than in the hearts of non-alcoholic subjects (Kesteloot et al., 1968; Morin and Daniel, 1967) (Table 8.4).

TABLE 8.3. NUTRIENT DEFICIENCIES AND EXCESSES ASSOCIATED WITH ALCOHOLIC HEART DISEASE

Disease	Nutrient deficiency or excess
Cardiac beri-beri	Thiamin deficiency
Alcoholic cardiomyopathy (with arythmia)	Potassium depletion
Beer drinkers' heart	Cobalt intoxication

NUTRITIONAL ASPECTS OF BONE DISEASE IN ALCOHOLICS

In 1965, Saville first demonstrated loss of bone mass in autopsy specimens obtained from alcoholics. In a 1975 paper on bone disease in alcoholics, Saville hypothesizes that alcohol abuse may be associated both with osteoporosis and an increased risk of fracture from mild to moderate trauma, particularly in relation to the hip, wrist, upper humorus and spine. In addition, a syndrome of non-traumatic osteonecrosis of the hip occurs with greater frequency in alcoholics; this condition being caused by a block of end arteries in the bone by fat emboli.

There are many factors which can contribute to the development of bone disease in alcoholics. Due to inebriation, the alcoholic stands at risk for sustaining falls and fractures. Alcoholics who develop recurrent peptic ulcers are more likely to be treated by partial gastrectomy than non-alcoholics, because they are unable to adhere to a medical regimen and diet. Nilsson and Weslin (1972) studied the bone-mineral mass in the distal end of the femur in 121 men, half of whom were alcoholics. It was shown that in the alcoholics, the bone mass was significantly decreased but only in those who had had a previous partial gastrectomy. The implication is that alcoholics who have had partial gastrectomy may develop post-gastrectomy bone disease. After gastrectomy, absorption of vitamin D and calcium may be reduced. Steatorrhea is frequently associated with post-gastrectomy bone disease, and it has been suggested that unabsorbed fatty acids may combine with calcium to impair absorption. However, attempts to demonstrate vitamin D malabsorption in post-gastrectomy patients have not yielded definitive evidence of vitamin D malabsorption. In spite of this negative finding with respect to vitamin D absorption, both radiological and biochemical studies of patients with post-gastrectomy bone disease have indicated presence both of osteoporosis and osteomalacia (Clark *et al.*, 1964; Alexander Williams, 1965).

Nilsson and Weslin reported in 1973 on associations between characteristics of alcoholics and the presence of bone disease. As in their earlier studies, their method of identifying osteoporosis was by measurement of the mineral content in both forearms, by the method of gamma-absorbtiometry. They found in young alcoholics that bone mass did not differ from that found in a control population. However, there was an association between age and mineral thickness in both the alcoholic and control groups, such that in patients coming from a department for the treatment of alcoholism, and in those coming from an orthopedic department, there was a progressive decrease in the mineral thickness of the arm with age, which the authors considered could reflect the duration of alcoholism. As in the previous study by these investigators, partial gastrectomy had been carried out in a number of the alcoholic cases. If the operated cases were removed from the comparisons of bone mineral mass, there was still a reduction in bone mineral mass in the alcoholics as compared to the control subjects.

A possible further insight into the etiology of bone disease in alcoholics, or at least in alcoholics with cirrhosis, has been obtained by Hepner and Roginsky (1975). During a protein binding assay these investigators studied the serum levels of 25 hydroxycholecalciferol (25-OHD) and 20 healthy control subjects, 31 cirrhotics who had stopped drinking within 6 months of the study, 8 alcoholic cirrhotics and also 15 alcoholics without cirrhosis of whom the latter 2 groups were still drinking. Also, parenteral dosages of vitamin D$_3$ (120 μg) was administered to 5 control subjects and 6 non-alcoholic cirrhotics, and the serum 25-OHD was again determined 24 hrs later. Serum levels of 25-OHD were significantly lower in the non-alcoholic cirrhotics than in the "control subjects," and also in the alcoholic (actively drinking) cirrhotics. The alcoholics who had normal liver function also had serum OHD levels within the limits of the normal controls. Serum-25-OHD levels in the non-alcoholic cirrhotics was correlated with serum albumin values. It increased significantly in the 5 control subjects after vitamin D$_3$ had been administered, and there was no similar rise in the level of 25-OHD in the non-alcoholic cirrhotics. It is suggested that the 25-hydroxylation of vitamin D in the liver is impaired in cirrhosis, and that perhaps this impairment may be due to liver abnormalities rather than alcohol consumption per se. A further suggestion is that metabolic bone disease may be related to the hydroxylation defect of vitamin D in cirrhotic patients.

In several reports from South Africa, descriptions have been given of Bantu patients with a history of alcoholism who showed evidence of iron storage disease, osteoporosis, and scurvy (Charlton et al., 1973).

Observations have previously been made in the U.S. of an impaired vitamin C status of alcoholics who were hospitalized. However, no studies were conducted with respect to the incidence or severity of bone disease in these ascorbic acid deficient patients (Lester et al., 1960).

Evidence has been presented that siderosis or iron overload directly influences ascorbic acid metabolism. The ferric iron accelerates oxidative catabolism of ascorbic acid in vitro, and it has been suggested that when there are deposits of ferric iron in the tissues, such as may occur in patients with siderosis or hemochromatosis, that a similar rapid breakdown of ascorbic acid may occur (Schulz and Swanepoel, 1962).

Scorbutic patients with severe siderosis have an increased urinary output of oxalic acid, the oxidation end product of ascorbic acid, after the vitamin is administered (Lynch et al., 1967a; Lynch et al., 1967b). In scorbutic guinea pigs, decreased bone formation and increased bone resorption have been found. The syndrome of siderosis, scurvy and osteoporosis was induced in guinea pigs by Wapnick et al. (1971), who produce iron overload by injecting iron dextran and maintaining the animals on their normal daily requirement of ascorbic acid. Both the osteoporosis and the scurvy could be prevented by giving large supplements of ascorbic acid by the parenteral route.

In Bantu subjects with iron overload, scurvy and osteoporosis, evidence has been obtained through experiments involving intravenous injections of radiolabelled calcium, that there is decreased bone formation and increased bone resorption. It has further been demonstrated that when these patients are given large doses of ascorbic acid, urinary calcium excretion is diminished.

Wapnick et al. (1970) showed that ascorbic acid deficiency affects iron metabolism. There has been some evidence to suggest that, in scurvy, the release of iron from reticuloendothelial stores may be impaired (Lipschutz et al., 1971).

Whereas present information allows us to identify several causes and causal relationships between the occurrence of bone disease and alcoholism, and to conclude that causes may be nutritional, it is equally clear that bone disease in alcoholics is multifactorial and that there are several types. As with other nutritional syndromes in alcoholics, impaired utilization of nutrients which contribute to the development of bone disease is secondary to the direct effects of ethanol. It has been demonstrated that aberrant nutrient utilization can contribute both to development of osteoporosis and osteomalacia in alcoholics (Table 8.4).

TABLE 8.4 NUTRITIONAL DISORDERS AND ALCOHOLIC BONE DISEASE.

Disease complex	Nutrient deficiency or excess
Postgastrectomy Osteomalacia/ Osteoporosis	Vitamin D and calcium malabsorption
Osteomalacia in cirrhosis	Hepatic defect in vitamin D metabolism
Bantu osteoporosis	Vitamin C deficiency Iron Overload

NUTRITIONAL DISEASE IN ALCOHOLIC CIRRHOSIS

Mortality from cirrhosis of the liver has been increasing in the United States for a number of years. According to a recent report in the Metropolitan Statistical Bulletin (1977), cirrhosis accounts for 33,000 deaths a year, and ranks seventh among leading causes of death in the country. Increases and reported mortality from cirrhosis are attributed both to improved methods of diagnosis and reporting on death certificates. We would assume that changes in the mortality from cirrhosis also affect changes in the incidence of alcoholism, though the latter now, as in the past, is grossly underreported. Although it is generally acknowledged that Laennec's cirrhosis is a common chronic liver disease in alcoholics, the question remains why some alcoholics develop cirrhosis and others do not. Rubin and Popper (1967) indicated that the definition of cirrhosis remained controversial. These authors divide cirrhosis into two types: monolobular and multilobular cirrhosis; the former being synonymous with Laennec's cirrhosis, as seen in alcoholics. In this disease the major change in the liver consists in the presence of connective tissue septa involving all portal tracts.

In the rat, cirrhosis has been produced by dietary choline deficiency (Best et al., 1949; Hartroft and Ridout, 1971; Hartroft and Grisham, 1960). These findings in experimental animals led to the extrapolation to human subjects with the result that it was inferred that alcoholic cirrhosis could also develop because of a dietary deficiency of lipotropic factors. Support for a primary nutritional etiology of alcoholic cirrhosis is not strong at the present time. Indeed, Klatskin, in 1961, focused attention on the role of ethanol per se in the development of cirrhosis.

Isselbacher and Greenberger (1964) comment that in patients with Laennec's cirrhosis, the discontinuation of alcohol abuse often leads to significant clinical improvements. These authors also note that cirrhosis can develop, whether or not dietary intake of nutrients is adequate.

Rubin and Lieber (1974) showed that the whole spectrum of alcoholic liver injury including cirrhosis could be produced in baboons consuming large amounts of alcohol for long periods with a nutritionally adequate diet. While the nutritional adequacy of the diet fed to these primates has been disputed, because of increased nutrient requirements imposed by the drug, no specific nutrient deficiency in man or subhuman primates has been shown to produce the histological picture of alcoholic cirrhosis.

Nevertheless, cirrhosis of the liver in alcoholics is associated with malnutrition. The prevalence of hypovitaminemia in cirrhotic patients was reported by Leevy et al. (1970). As reflected by reduced circulating vitamin levels, the commonest deficiencies were of folic acid, followed by vitamin B6, and thiamin. Their patients showed these biochemical evidences of hypovitaminosis, although they received therapeutic multivitamin capsules daily. The clinical signs of vitamin deficiency included glossitis, peripheral neuropathy, and macrocytic anemia. These authors indicate that there may be a "malutilization of vitamins" in cirrhosis, as in other diseases associated with hepatic dysfunction, and that also vitamin storage in the liver is impaired. They cite studies indicating that in cirrhosis there is an 80% reduction in the total liver content of niacin, a 60% reduction in the liver level of vitamin B12 and folacin, and a 50% reduction in vitamin B6. They also entertain the concept that vitamin requirements are increased in order to effect tissue damage and also to compensate for depressed hepatic storage capacity.

Reduction in the liver content of specific vitamins does not, of course, imply failure to store these nutrients, but may also be related to decreased intake or malabsorption. Klipstein and Lindenbaum (1965) explain that when megaloblastic anemia occurs in patients with alcoholic cirrhosis, there is usually a history of poor dietary intake of folic acid. These authors mention the work of Cherrick et al. (1965), who proposed that in cirrhosis the liver may be unable to take up this vitamin.

Urinary folacin losses have been found to be increased in cirrhosis, and Retief and Huskisson (1969), who carried out these studies, suggest that hyperexcretion of folacin may contribute to the development of deficiency of the vitamin in chronic liver disease.

Single or multiple B vitamin deficiencies are commonly seen in alcoholics with cirrhosis or evidence of B vitamin depletion has been obtained by biochemical methods. Rosenthal et al. (1973) obtained biochemical evidence of riboflavin deficiency in 11 out of 22 alcoholic patients who required hospitalization for alcoholic diseases, including alcoholic liver disease. Evidence of riboflavin deficiency was obtained from erythrocyte glutathione reductase assays. Although it is tempting to suggest that, in alcoholics with cirrhosis, there might be an impairment in the conversion of riboflavin to the coenzyme forms, this is not investigated in the study cited.

Labadarios et al. (1976) found in 32 patients with decompensated cirrhosis, a 29% incidence of thiamin deficiency and an 88% incidence of a deficiency of vitamin B6. They also found in the same group a 14% incidence of ascorbic acid deficiency. A similar incidence of vitamin deficiencies was found in a group of patients with non-alcoholic liver disease. When pharmacologic doses of thiamin and ascorbic acid were given by the intravenous route, deficiencies of these vitamins were corrected, but when 50 mg and 100 mg of pyridoxine hydrochloride was given intravenously, plasma levels of pyridoxal phosphate increased to normal values in only 33% of the alcoholic patients. On the other hand, administration of pyridoxal-5-phosphate resulted in an increase in plasma pyridoxal phosphate levels. It is suggested by these investigators that there may be an increased rate of degradation of, or elimination of, pyridoxal phosphate in patients with cirrhosis, although they also suggest that perhaps the conversion of pyridoxine to pyridoxal phosphate may be impaired. Again, the possibility is raised that the pyridoxal phosphate deficiency could be related to leakage of the vitamin from the damaged hepatocytes, though this would seem less likely in patients with cirrhosis.

Sorrell et al. showed that when rat liver is perfused with ethanol, this causes a release of many vitamins from liver stores, including vitamin B_{12}, vitamin B_6, panthothenate, thiamin, riboflavin, niacin, and folacin. Although we may assume that many patients with cirrhosis continue in alcohol abuse, it cannot be assumed that B vitamin deficiencies in these patients are due to such washing-out of vitamins from the alcohol damaged liver. More work is required to define the metabolic consequences of cirrhosis, with respect to biotransformation of vitamins.

It is common for chronic alcoholics with Laennec's cirrhosis to be sterile and to show other evidence of impaired gonadal function. Signs of hypogonadism include testicular atrophy, impotence, decreased beard and pubic hair, and reduced prostatic size. Gynecomastia may also be present but is an inconsistent feature of the syndrome (Barr and Som, 1957; Bennett et al., 1950; Lloyd and Williams, 1948).

Van Thiel et al. (1974a) studied causal mechanisms responsible for hypogonadism in men with alcoholic liver disease. They identified both a primary gonadal failure and also hypothalamic-pituitary suppression, which could be responsible for the observed combination of feminization and testicular dysfunction.

Van Thiel et al. (1974b) also studied the nutritional implications of testicular atrophy in alcoholics. They noted that in their own previous studies they have found a high incidence of azoospermia, not only in patients with Laennec's cirrhosis, but also in other alcoholics with milder liver disease. They also mention studies of a high incidence of nightblindness among alcoholics. Association of nightblindness and testicular failure suggests a relative vitamin A deficiency, since this vitamin is required both for spermatogenesis and also for visual function. Alcohol dehydrogenase, one of the enzymes necessary for ethanol oxidation, is also required for the conversion of retinol to retinal by testicular tissue. Employing tissues obtained from experimental rats, it was shown by these investigators that ethanol inhibits the oxidation of retinol by testicular homogenates which contain alcohol dehydrogenase A suggestion is made that in alcoholics the competitive utilization of alcohol dehydrogenase for the metabolism of ethanol and for the metabolism of vitamin A to its active form, causes a functional disturbance in vitamin A-dependent systems.

Earlier studies by Mezey and Holt (1971) suggested that both ethanol and retinol are oxidized by the same enzyme in the liver, but not in the retina. They indicate that data have been obtained that with both ethanol and retinol as substrates, differential activity of the isoenzymes of human alcohol dehydrogenase may be obtained for the liver and retinal tissues.

Some of the nutritional disturbances found in cirrhotics may be the result of heavy ethanol ingestion rather than due to hepatic dysfunction. Sullivan and Lankford (1965) showed that in chronic alcoholics, decreased serum zinc concentrations are associated with hyperzincuria, an increased renal clearance of zinc. They noted that in most patients, the hyperzincuria is only transient and that zinc excretion returns to normal following a short period of abstinence. They do, however, indicate that in cirrhotic patients a true zinc deficiency may occur.

Liver alcohol dehydrogenase contains 4 zinc atoms per mole of enzyme. It was shown by Weiner (1969) that when zinc is removed from the enzyme, the apoenzyme is catalytically inactive.

Florid cases of zinc deficiency have also been encountered among alcoholics with cirrhosis. Acquired alcoholic zinc deficiency as well as non-alcohol acquired zinc deficiency present with erythroderma or a psoriasiform dermatosis, anorexia, and if trauma or surgery has been recent, by poor wound healing. Reported cases are few, and patients usually have other nutritional deficiencies including protein deficiency with hypoproteinemia. History was typical in a case recently seen by the author for the establishment of diagnosis. A male alcoholic with cirrhosis had been admitted to hospital with rectal carcinoma which was resected. During a period of intravenous fluid administration in the immediate post-surgical period, he developed a generalized dermatosis, beginning on the trunk and arms, and spreading to other parts of the body. His operation wounds failed to heal. When intravenous fluids were discontinued he complained about the tastelessness of the food in the hospital. Laboratory studies including serum zinc levels reported a diagnosis of zinc deficiency, as well as hypoalbuminemia. His clinical condition responded to administration of zinc sulfate orally (Roe, unpublished).

SELECTED REFERENCES

Alexander, C.S. 1966. Idiopathic heart disease. Analysis of 100 cases, with special reference to chronic alcoholism. Amer. J. Med. 41: 213-227.

Alexander, L. 1940. Wernicke's disease. Amer. J. Path. 16: 61-70.

Alexander W.J. 1965. The long-term effects of partial gastrectomy. IN *Recent Advances in Gastroenterology*. Eds. Badenoch, J. and Brooke, B.N. J & A Churchill Ltd., London. 86-106.

Anderson, B.B., Saary, M., Stephens, A.D., Perry, G.M., Lersundi, I.C. and Horn, J.E. 1976. Effect of riboflavin on red-cell metabolism of vitamin B6. Nature 264: 574-575.

Barr, R.W. and Som, S.C. 1957. Endocrine abnormalities accompanying hepatic cirrhosis and hepatoma. J. Clin. Endocrin. Metab. 17: 1017-1029.

Bennett, H.S., Baggenstoss, A.H. and Butt, H.R. 1950. Testes, breast and prostate of men who die of cirrhosis of liver. Amer. J. Clin. Pathol. 20: 814-828.

Best, C.H., Hartroft, W.S., Lucas, C.C. and Ridout, J.H. 1949. Liver damage produced by feeding alcohol or sugar and its prevention by choline. Brit. Med. J. 2: 1001-1006.

Bianco, A. and Jolliffe, N. 1938. The anemia of alcohol addicts. Observations as to the role of liver disease, achlorhydria, nutritional factors and alcohol on its production. Amer. J. Med. Sci. 196: 414-420.

Bing, R.J., Tillman, H. and Ikeda, S. 1975. Metabolic effects of alcohol on the heart. IN Medical Consequences of Alcoholism. Ann. New York Acad. Sci. 252: 243-249.

Blass, J.P. and Gibson, G.E. 1977. Abnormalities of a thiamin-requiring enzyme in patients with Wernicke-Korsakoff syndrome. New Eng. J. Med. 297: 1367-1370.

Brigden, W. and Robinson, J. 1964. Alcoholic heart disease. Brit. Med. J. 2: 1283-1289.

Chanarin, I. 1969. *The Megaloblastic Anemias*. Blackwell Scientific Publ., Oxford.

Charlton, R.W., Bothwell, T.H. and Seftel, H.C. 1973. Dietary iron overload. Clin. Haematol. 2: 383-403.

Clark, C.G., Crooks, J., Dawson, A. and Mitchell, P.E.G. 1964. Disordered calcium metabolism after Polya partial gastrectomy. Lancet 1: 734-738.

Demakis, J.G., Proskey, A., Rahimtoola, S.H., Sutton, G.C., Rosen, K.M., Gunnar, R.M. and Tobin, J.R. 1974. The natural course of alcoholic cardiomyopathy. Ann. Intern. Med. 80: 293-297.

Douglas Talbott, G. 1975. Primary alcoholic heart disease. IN Medical Consequences of Alcoholism. Ann. New York Acad. Sci. 252: 237-242.

Eichner, E.R., Buchanon, B., Smith, J.W. and Hillman, R.S. 1972. Variations in the hematologic and medical status of alcoholics. Amer. J. Med. Sci. 263: 35-42.

Eichner, E.R. and Hillman, H.S. 1971. The evolution of anemia in alcoholic patients. Amer. J. Med. 50: 218-232.

Eichner, E.R. and Hillman, R.S. 1973. Effect of alcohol on serum folate level. J. Clin. Invest. 52: 584-591.

Eichner, E.R., Pierce, H.I. and Hillman, R.S. 1971. Folate balance in dietary-induced megaloblastic anemia. New Eng. J. Med. 28: 933-938.

Evans, C.A., Carlson, W.E. and Green, R.G. 1942. The pathology of Chastek paralysis in foxes. Amer. J. Path. 18: 79-92.

Feuerlein, W. 1977. Neuropsychiatric disorders of alcoholism. Second Europ. Nutrit. Conf., Munich, 1976, Nutr. Metab. 21: 163-174.

Flink, E.B. 1971. Mineral metabolism in alcoholism. IN *The Biology of Alcoholism*, Vol. 1. Biochemistry. Eds. Kissin, B. and Begleiter, H. Plenum Press, New York, London. pp. 378-386.

Goldsmith, G.A. 1975. Riboflavin deficiency. IN *Riboflavin*. Ed. Rivlin, R. S., Plenum Press, New York and London. p. 228.

Hartroft, W.S. and Grisham, J.W. 1960. Cirrhosis of "post-necrotic" type in choline deficient rats. Fed. Proc. 19: 186.

Hartroft, W.S. and Ridout, J.H. 1951. Pathogenesis of the cirrhosis produced by choline deficiency. Escape of lipid from fatty hepatic cysts into the biliary and vascular systems. Amer. J. Path. 27: 951-990.

Hepner, G.W. and Roginsky, M. 1975. Abnormal metabolism of vitamin D. in patients with cirrhosis. Clin. Res. 23: 322A, abs.

Herbert, V., Zalusky, R. and Davidson, C.S. 1963. Correlation of folate deficiency with alcoholism and associated macrocytosis, anemia, and liver disease. Ann. Intern. Med. 58: 977-987.

Hillman, R.S. 1975. Alcohol and hematopoiesis. IN Medical Consequences of Alcoholism. Ann. New York Acad. Sci. 252: 297-306.

Hines, J.D. 1975. Hematologic abnormalities involving vitamin B_6 and folate metabolism in alcoholic subjects. IN Medical Consequences of Alcoholism. Ann. New York Acad. Sci. 252: 316-327.

Hines, H.D. and Cowan, D.H. 1970. Studies on the pathogenesis of alcohol-induced sideroblastic bone-marrow abnormalities. New Eng. J. Med. 283: 441-446.

Hourihane, D.O'B. and Weir, D.G. 1970. Suppression of erythropoiesis by alcohol. Brit. Med. J. 1: 86-89.

Hunter, J.M. 1976. Hypothermia and Wernicke's encephalopathy. Brit. Med. J. 2: 563-564.

Isselbacher, J. and Greenberger, N.J. 1964. Metabolic effects of alcohol on the liver. New Eng. J. Med. 270: 351-410.

Itokawa, Y. and Cooper, J.R. 1970. Ion movements and thiamin, II. The release of the vitamin from membrane fragments. Biochem. Biophys. Acta 196: 274-284.

Jandl, J.H. 1955. The anemia of liver disease: Observations on its mechanism. J. Clin. Invest. 34: 390-404.

Jolliffe, N., Wortis, H. and Fein, H.D. 1941. The Wernicke syndrome. Arch. Neurol. Psychiat. 46: 569-597.

Jubb, K.V., Saunders, L.Z. and Coates, H.V. 1956. Thiamine deficiency encephalopathy in cats. J. Comp. Pathol. 66: 217-227.

Kesteloot, H., Roelandt, J., Willems, J., Claes, J.H. and Joussens, J. V. 1968. An inquiry into the role of cobalt in the heart disease of chronic beer drinkers. Circulation 37: 854-864.

Klatskin, G. 1961. Alcohol and its relation to liver damage. Gastroenterology 41: 443-451.

Klipstein, F.A. and Lindenbaum, J. 1965. Folate deficiency in chronic liver disease. Blood 25: 443-455.

Kondi, A. and Foy, H. 1964. Vacuolization of early erythroblasts in riboflavin deficient baboons and in marasmus and kwashiorkor. Lancet 2: 1157.

Labadarios, D., Rossouw, J.E., Davis, M. and Williams, R. 1976. Pyridoxine deficiency in severe liver disease. Proc. Nutr. Soc. 35: 141A.

Lane, F., Goff, P., McGuffin, R., Eichner, E.R. and Hillman, R.S. 1976. Folic acid metabolism in normal, folate deficient and alcoholic man. Brit. J. Haematol. 34: 489-500.

Lester, D., Buccino, R. and Bizzocco, D. 1960. The vitamin C status of alcoholics. J. Nutr. 70: 278-282.

Leevy, C.M., Thompson, A. and Baker, H. 1970. Vitamins and liver injury. Amer. J. Clin. Nutr. 23: 493-499.

Lhermitte, F., Marteau, R., Serdaru, M. and Chedru, F. 1977. Signs of interhemispheric disconnection in Marchiafava-Bignami disease. Arch. Neurol. 34: 254.

Lindenbaum, J. and Lieber, C.S. 1969. Hematologic effects of alcohol in man in the absence of nutritional deficiency. New Eng. J. Med. 281: 333-338.

Lipschitz, D.A., Bothwell, T.H., Seftel, H.C., Wapnick, A.A. and Charlton, R. W. 1971. The role of ascorbic acid in the metabolism of storage iron. Brit. J. Haematol. 20: 155-163.

Lloyd, C.W. and Williams, R.H. 1948. Endocrine changes associated with Laennec's cirrhosis of the liver. Amer. J. Med. 4: 315-330.

Lumeng, L. and Li, T-K. 1974. Vitamin B6 metabolism in chronic alcohol abuse. Pyridoxal phosphate levels in plasma, and the effects of acetaldehyde on pyridoxal phosphate synthesis and degradation in human erythrocytes. J. Clin. Invest. 53: 693-704.

Lynch, S.R., Berelowitz, I., Seftel, H.C., Miller, G.B., Krawitz, P., Charlton, R. W. and Bothwell, T.H. 1967a. Osteoporosis in Johannesburg Bantu males. Its relationship to siderosis and ascorbic acid deficiency. Amer. J. Clin. Nutr. 20: 799-807.

Lynch, S.R., Seftel, H.C., Torance, J.D., Charlton, R.W. and Bothwell, T. H. 1967b. Accelerated oxidative catabolism of ascorbic acid in siderotic Bantu. Amer. J. Clin. Nutr. 20: 641-647.

McDonald, C.D., Burch, G.E. and Walsh, J.J. 1971. Alcoholic cardiomyopathy managed by prolonged bed rest. Ann. Intern. Med. 74: 581-591.

Metropolitan Statistical Bulletin 58: 1977. Recent Trends in Mortality from Cirrhosis of the Liver. 9-11.

Mezey, E. and Holt, P.R. 1971. The inhibitory effect of ethanol on retinol oxidation by human liver and cattle. Retina Exp. Molec. Pathol. 15: 148-156.

Morin, Y. and Daniel, P.1967. Quebec beer drinkers' cardiomyopathy. Etiological considerations. Canad. Med. Assn. J. 97: 926, 1967; Canad. Med. Assn. Symp., Quebec beer drinkers' cardiomyopathy, Canad. Med. Assn. J. 97: 881-931.

Nilsson, B.E. and Weslin, N.E. 1972. Femur density in alcoholism and after gastrectomy. Calc. Tiss. Res. 10: 167-170.

Nilsson, B.E. and Weslin, N.E. 1973. Changes in bone mass in alcoholics. Clin. Orthopaed. Rel. Res. 90: 229-232. Ed. Urist, M.R., J.B. Lippincott Co., Phila.

Pincus, J.H., Cooper, J.R., Murphy, J.V., Rabe, E.F., Lonsoale, D. and Dunne, H. G. 1973. Thiamine derivatives in subacute necrotizing encephalomyelopathy. A preliminary report. Pediatrics 51: 716-721.

Platt, B.S. and Lu, G.D. 1939. Studies on metabolism of pyruvic acid in normal and vitamin B_1-deficient states; accumulation of pyruvic acid and other carbonyl compounds in beriberi and effect of vitamin B_1. Biochem. J. 33: 1525-1537.

Reed, D.H., Jolly, R.D. and Alley, M.R. 1977. Polio encephalomalacia of dogs with thiamine deficiency. Vet. Pathol. 14: 103-112.

Retief, F.P. and Huskisson, Y.J. 1969. Serum and urinary folate in liver disease. Brit. Med. J. 2: 150-153.

Riggs, H.E. and Boles, R.S. 1944-45. Wernicke's disease. A clinical and pathological study of 42 cases. Quart. J. Stud. Alcohol 5: 361-370.

Rinehart, J.F., Friedman, M. and Greenberg, L.D. 1949. Effect of experimental thiamine deficiency on the nervous system of the rhesus monkey. Arch. Path. 48: 129-139.

Rosenbach, L.M., Caviles, A.P. and Mitus, W.J. 1960. Chloramphenicol toxicity: Reversible vacuolization of erythroid cells. New Eng. J. Med. 263: 724-728.

Rosenthal, W.S., Adham, N.F., Lopez, R. and Cooperman, J.M. 1973. Riboflavin deficiency in complicated chronic alcoholism. Amer. J. Clin. Nutr. 26: 858-860.

Rubin, E., Katz, A.M., Lieber, C.S., Stein, E.P. and Puszkin, S. 1976. Muscle damage produced by chronic alcohol consumption. Amer. J. Path. 83: 499-512.

Rubin, E. and Lieber, C.S. 1974. Fatty liver, alcoholic hepatitis, and cirrhosis produced by alcohol in primates. New Eng. J. Med. 290: 120-135.

Rubin, E. and Popper, H. 1967. The evolution of human cirrhosis deduced from observations in experimental animals. Medicine 46: 163-183.

Sauberlich, H.E. 1967. Biochemical alterations in thiamin deficiency—their interpretation. Amer. J. Clin. Nutr. 20: 528-546.

Saville, P.D. 1965. Changes in bone mass with age and alcoholism. J. Bone Joint Surg. 47-A: 492-499.

Saville, P.D. 1975. Alcohol-related skeletal disorders. IN Medical Consequences of Alcoholism. Ann. New York Acad. Sci. 252: 286-291.

Schulz, E.J. and Swanepoel, H. 1962. Scorbutic pseudoscleroderma. An aspect of Bantu siderosis. South African Med. J. 36: 367-372.

Schwartz, L., Sample, K.A. and Wigle, E.D. 1975. Severe alcoholic cardiomyopathy reversed with abstention from alcohol. Amer. J. Cardiol. 36: 963-966.

Sherman, J.D., Greenfield, J.B. and Ingall, D. 1964. Reversible bone-marrow vacuolizations in phenylketonuria. New Eng. J. Med. 270: 810-814.

Sinclair, H.M. 1972. Nutritional aspects of alcohol consumption. Proc. Nutr. Soc. 31: 117-122.

Sorrell, M.F., Baker, H., Barak, A.J. and Frank, O. 1974. Release by ethanol of vitamins into rat liver perfusates. Amer. J. Clin. Nutr. 27: 743-745.

Sullivan, J.F., Parker, M. and Carson, S.B. 1968. Tissue cobalt in "beer drinkers" myocardiopathy. J. Lab. Clin. Med. 71: 893-896.

Sullivan, J.F. and Lankford, H.G. 1965. Zinc metabolism and chronic alcoholism. Amer. J. Clin. Nutr. 17: 57-63.

Tanphaichitr, V. 1976. Thiamin. IN *Present Knowledge in Nutrition*, 4th ed. Nutrition Foundation, Inc., New York, Washington. pp. 141-148.

Thomson, A.D., Baker, H. and Leevy, C.M. 1970. Patterns of ^{35}S-thiamine hydrochloride absorption in the malnourished alcoholic patient. J. Lab. Clin. Med. 76: 34-45.

Tomasulo, P.A., Kater, M.H. and Iber, F.L. 1968. Impairment of thiamin absorption in alcoholism. Amer. J. Clin. Nutr. 21: 1340-1344.

Van Itallie, T.B. and Follis, R.H. Jr. 1974. Thiamin deficiency, ariboflavinosis, and vitamin B6 deficiency. IN *Harrison's Principles of Internal Medicine*, 7th ed., Eds. Wintrobe, M., Thorn, G.W., Adams, R.D. et al. McGraw-Hill, New York. 430-433.

Van Thiel, D.H., Lester, R. and Sherins, R.J. 1974a. Hypogonadism in alcoholic liver disease: evidence for a double defect. Gastroenterology 67: 1188-1199.

Van Thiel, D.H., Gavaler, J. and Lester, R. 1974b. Ethanol inhibition of vitamin A metabolism in the testes: possible mechanism for sterility in alcoholics. Science 186: 941-942.

Vetter, W.R., Cohn, L.H. and Reichgott, J. 1967. Hypokalemia and electro-cardiographic abnormalities during acute alcohol withdrawal. Arch. Intern. Med. 120: 536-540.

Victor, M., Adams, R.D. and Collins, G.H. 1971. The Wernicke-Korsakoff syndrome. A clinical and pathological study of 245 patients, 82 with post-mortem examination. F.A. Davis Co., Philadelphia.

Victor, M., Altschule, M.D. and Holliday, P.D. et al. 1957. Carbohydrate metabolism in brain disease. VIII. Carbohydrate metabolism in Wernicke's encephalopathy associated with alcoholism. Arch. Intern. Med. 99: 28-39.

Wada, H. and Snell, E.E. 1961. The enzymatic oxidation of pyridoxine and pyridoxamine phosphates. J. Biochem. 236: 2089-2095.

Wapnik, A.A., Bothwell, T.H. and Seftel, H. 1970. The relationship between iron levels and ascorbic acid stores in siderotic Bantu. Brit. J. Haematol. 19: 271-276.

Wapnik, A.A., Lynch, S.R., Seftel, H.C., Charlton, R.W., Bothwell, T.H. and Jowsey, J. 1971. The effect of siderosis and ascorbic acid depletion on bone metabolism, with special reference to osteoporosis in the Bantu. Brit. J. Nutr. 25: 367-376.

Weiner, H. 1969. The role of zinc in liver alcohol dehydrogenase. IN *Biochemical and Clinical Aspects of Alcohol Metabolism*. Ed. Sardesai, V.M. Charles C. Thomas Co., Springfield Illinois. 29-33.

Wu, A., Chanarin, I., and Levi, A.J. 1974. Macrocytosis of chronic alcoholism. Lancet 1: 829-830.

Zimmerman, H. M. 1939. The pathology of the nervous system in vitamin deficiencies. Yale J. Biomed. 12: 23-28.

9

Nutritional Assessment of Alcoholics

Nutritional assessment of alcoholics is an essential prerequisite for dietary prescription, for estimation of compliance with dietary advice, for determination of nutrient requirements prior to surgery, and in gauging the risks of therapeutic drugs. The components of the assessment are the nutritional history and the evaluation of current nutritional status. A complete nutritional assessment facilitates appropriate intervention and significantly improves outcome. However, the feasibility of such an assessment is limited by lack of patient cooperation, by the urgency of treatment, by the lack of clinical nutritionists or dietitians with the skills necessary to obtain a meaningful dietary history, and by lack of a laboratory facility where biochemical assessment of nutritional status can be carried out.

DIETARY METHODOLOGY

Dietary methodology should be selected on the basis of goals and circumstances. When the aim is a complete nutritional assessment and the patient or patient's family are able to supply reliable information, then a diet history of the Burke (1947) type should be taken which includes past as well as present food intake, food intolerances, food preferences and dislikes, cultural and religious influence on foods consumed, medical problems which have interfered with food intake, and socioeconomic factors as well as living conditions which influence ability to obtain, store and prepare food (Eagles and Longman, 1963).

Alternative methods of dietary methodology can be explored to determine current energy and nutrient intake including intake of alcoholic beverages and food and nutrient supplements. Single 24-hour recalls of intake should be avoided since they may not be representative of the accustomed eating pattern. The patient may not remember what

149

s/he ate or drank in the last 24 hours because of inebriation or through a desire to please or impress the interrogator, may give a false record. Repeated 24-hour recalls are more satisfactory as records of prevailing patterns of intake and the quality of these records can be improved when the patient's recall is assisted by input from family members or friends.

Three, five or seven day diet diaries usually provide reasonably quantitative information on the diet. Selection of the duration of the diet diary must depend on the judgement of the nutritionists or physicians with respect to the patient's ability to retain interest in keeping the record. It is essential that the patient be instructed as to how to record intake with special emphasis on the time and place where food is consumed, and on the inclusion of quantitative information. It has been our experience that seven-day diet diaries are superior to three or five day diaries, particularly when the respondent is a binge drinker who, for example, only drinks heavily 1-3 days a week and on those days only consumes very little food.

Food frequency records are useful if the aim is to examine the quality of the diet. Semi-quantitative information can be added to the food frequency form particularly with regard to food and beverage items which are taken daily. Examples of appropriate forms to be used for 24-hour recall, diet history, diet diary, and food frequency records, are shown in Tables 9.1A to 9.1D.

Underreporting of alcohol intake is common, and may be due to the patients' diffidence or memory loss, or to the lack of explanation by the interrogator as to the desired method for expressing intake. Whatever dietary method is selected, it is desirable to collect information on the type of beverage, the amount, and the frequency of intake. The patient should be advised that this can be expressed as glasses with detail on the size of the glass or as cans of beer or bottles of wine or liquor. If the patient is drinking directly out of a bottle, the amount remaining in the bottle at the end of the day may be recorded. When patients are drinking in bars or other public places ideally they may be assisted in estimating the amount consumed by the bartender.

All dietary records should include intake of nutrient supplements with information on the brand name and generic description.

Analysis of dietary records should be by a nutritionist who is familiar with the use of food composition tables, or who has access to a food composition data bank (Agricultural Handbook No. 456) which can be utilized in computer analysis. In the event that a physician or other non-nutritionist is collecting dietary information, analysis of a limited diet with respect to key nutrients can be obtained by using information

TABLE 9.1A. TWENTY-FOUR HOUR DIET RECALL METHOD

Instruction to nutritionist or other health care personnel obtaining information:
1. Oral recall by the patient preferred. Records should be made by the interrogator.
2. Recall data should be for 2 or more non-consecutive 24-hr. periods.
3. Method should not be used to obtain dietary information from individual patients unless validity can be checked by direct observation of 2 or more meals consumed which are then recalled (observation of patients' actual food consumption can be by a trained observer, family member, or friend).
4. Recall for volumes of beverages and portion sizes for food can be assisted by use of food models or picture cards.
5. Standard probing procedures should be employed to relate food intake to time, place, activity, and alcohol ingestion.
6. Recall should begin with the most recent meal eaten and work backwards for 24 hrs.
7. Records sheets should be completed under the following headings:

Name: Education (last grade completed):

Age:

Code No.:   Date/Time of Interview

Ingestion Period	Food Item	Amount Eaten	Beverage Item	Amount Drunk	Where Consumed

TABLE 9.1B. DIET HISTORY.

1. How many times a week do you eat the following meals or snacks?

Breakfast	0	1	2	3	4	5	6	7
Mid-morning snack	0	1	2	3	4	5	6	7
Lunch	0	1	2	3	4	5	6	7

Mid-afternoon snack	0	1	2	3	4	5	6	7
Dinner	0	1	2	3	4	5	6	7
Bedtime snack	0	1	2	3	4	5	6	7

2. How many times a week do you eat meals out?

Breakfast	0	1	2	3	4	5	6	7
Lunch	0	1	2	3	4	5	6	7
Dinner	0	1	2	3	4	5	6	7

3. Please indicate which of the following foods and beverages you eat
and how often. If you do not eat or drink these foods, indicate why:

Food or Beverage	Yes	No	If yes:	Daily	> once a week	< once a week
Milk						
Cheese						
Yogurt						
Ice cream						
Eggs						
Meat						
Cold cuts						
Fish						
Poultry						
Raw vegetables						
Cooked leafy green vegetables						
Cooked leafy yellow vegetables						
Beans						
Fruits						
Fruit juice						
Enriched bread						
Fortified breakfast cereals						
Peanut butter						

I do not drink/eat the following because:

Food or beverage	Dislike	Allergic	Gives diarrhea or other symptoms	Not on my diet	Too expensive	Cannot cook
Milk						
Cheese						
Yogurt						
Ice cream						
Eggs						
Meat						
Cold cuts						
Fish						
Poultry						
Raw vegetables						
Cooked leafy green vegetables						
Cooked leafy yellow vegetables						
Beans						
Fruits						
Fruit juice						
Enriched bread						
Fortified breakfast cereals						
Peanut butter						

4. Do you or the person who buys and prepares your meals have use of:

	Yes	No
a car	___	___
a working stove	___	___
a refrigerator	___	___
a freezer	___	___
a food storage area	___	___

5. Do you take vitamins, iron or tonics? Yes____ No____
If yes:

Proprietary Brand	Generic Name	Dose	Frequency	Duration

6. Are you on a special diet? Yes____ No____ If yes, for:
____ Allergy
____ Weight reduction
____ Liver disease
____ Diarrhea/constipation
____ Other (state):

7. How many days a week do you drink alcoholic beverages (please circle):

0   <1   1   2   3   4   5   6   7

8. On any drinking day, how many of the following drinks do you have? (1 drink of wine = 1 glass; 1 drink of beer = 1 can or bottle; 1 drink of liquor = 1 shot)

	Beer	Wine	Sherry	Whiskey	Gin	Vodka	Brandy	Rum	Other (state)
0									
1									
2									
3									
4									
5									
6									
7									
8									
9									
10									
>10									

Which of these drinks do you not consume? Beer____ Wine____
Sherry____ Whiskey____ Gin____ Vodka____ Brandy____
Rum____ Other (state):

9. How long does it take you to finish:

	< day	1 day	< week	> week
A six-pack of beer				
A half gallon of wine				
A quart of whiskey				
gin				
other liquor				

10. Please indicate which of the following non-alcoholic beverages you drink, and how often:

No. Times Per Week

	0	1	2	3	4	5	6	7	>7
Sodas									
Coffee									
Tea									

11. Do you eat candy? Yes_____ No_____ If yes, how many times per week?

0   1   2   3   4   5   6   7   >7

12. Do you smoke cigarettes? Yes_____ No_____ If yes, how often:

Occasionally   < pack   1-2 packs   2-3 packs   >3 packs
               per day   per day   per day   per day

TABLE 9.1C. DIET DIARY.

Date	Time	Place	Beverage or Food Item	Amount	Description
example: 8/10/78	9AM	Home	coffee, doughnut	1 cup	black sugar
	1PM	Bar	gin	4 shots	and tonic
	5 PM	Bar	gin	4 shots	Martinis
	6:30 PM	Home	gin Hamburger with bun	2 shots ½	Martinis MacDonald's
	10 PM	Home	Beer Popcorn	3 cans 1 cup	homemade

TABLE 9.1D.   FOOD FREQUENCY INTERVIEW

1. How many times per week do you consume (does your child consume):

Meat	0 1 2 3 4 5 6 7 >7 specify
Poultry	0 1 2 3 4 5 6 7 >7 specify
Fish	0 1 2 3 4 5 6 7 >7 specify
Hot dogs	0 1 2 3 4 5 6 7 >7 specify
Liver	0 1 2 3 4 5 6 7 >7 specify
Eggs	0 1 2 3 4 5 6 7 >7 specify
Cheese	0 1 2 3 4 5 6 7 >7 specify
Cottage cheese	0 1 2 3 4 5 6 7 >7 specify
Fruit juice	0 1 2 3 4 5 6 7 >7 specify
Raw fruit	0 1 2 3 4 5 6 7 >7 specify
Cooked fruit	0 1 2 3 4 5 6 7 >7 specify
Raw vegetables	0 1 2 3 4 5 6 7 >7 specify
Cooked green leafy vegetables	0 1 2 3 4 5 6 7 >7 specify
Beans and peas	0 1 2 3 4 5 6 7 >7 specify
Instant Breakfast	0 1 2 3 4 5 6 7 >7 specify
Peanut butter	0 1 2 3 4 5 6 7 >7 specify
Nuts	0 1 2 3 4 5 6 7 >7 specify
Doughnuts	0 1 2 3 4 5 6 7 >7 specify
Cereal breakfast foods	0 1 2 3 4 5 6 7 >7 specify
Crackers or pretzels	0 1 2 3 4 5 6 7 >7 specify
Macaroni, spaghetti, rice, noodles	0 1 2 3 4 5 6 7 >7 specify
Soft drinks	0 1 2 3 4 5 6 7 >7 specify
Coffee or tea	0 1 2 3 4 5 6 7 >7 specify
Beer	0 1 2 3 4 5 6 7 >7 specify
Wine	0 1 2 3 4 5 6 7 >7 specify
Liquor	0 1 2 3 4 5 6 7 >7 specify
Ice cream	0 1 2 3 4 5 6 7 >7 specify
Cookies	0 1 2 3 4 5 6 7 >7 specify
Pie, cake	0 1 2 3 4 5 6 7 >7 specify

2. How many servings per day do you eat of the following foods:

Bread, toast, rolls, muffins (1 slice or 1 item is a serving)	0 1 2 3 4 >4 specify
Milk—including addition to other foods (8 ounces is a serving)	0 1 2 3 4 >4 specify
Butter or margarine (1 tsp. is a serving)	0 1 2 3 4 >4 specify

INSTRUCTIONS TO INTERVIEWER:

Estimate frequency of food and beverage intake on the basis of food and drink groups.

1. Low frequency   =<7 times per week
    Intermediate frequency   = 7 times per week
    High frequency   =>7 times per week

2. Low frequency   =<4 times per day
    Intermediate frequency   = 4 times per day
    High frequency   =>4 times per day

Adjust frequency rating to age, sex, physiological status and activity of population group.

TABLE 9.2.   FOOD ENERGY AND NUTRIENT CONTENT OF SELECTED COMMON FOODS[2 ; 5]

Food	Amount[1]	Food energy kcal	Protein g	Fat g	Carbo-hydrate g	Calcium mg	Phosphorus mg	Iron mg	Sodium mg	Potassium mg	Vit. A IU	Thiamin mg	Riboflavin mg	Niacin mg	Ascorbic acid mg	Total Folacin µg	USDA Handbook No. 456 Ref. No.
Milk, whole	1 cup	159	8.5	8.5	12.0	288	277	0.1	122	251	350	0.07	0.41	0.2	2	10	1320b
Ice cream, vanilla	1 slice (⅛ qt.)	127	3.0	7.0	13.7	96	76		42	119	290	0.03	0.14	0.1	1	2	1139c
Bread, enriched, white	1 slice	76	2.4	0.9	14.1	24	27	0.7	142	29		0.07	0.06	0.7		3	461b
Bun, hamburger or Roll, frankfurter	1	119	3.3	2.2	21.2	30	34	0.3	202	38		0.02	0.04	0.3			1902c
Corn flakes, Frosted, fortified	1 cup	154	1.8	0.1	36.5	1.0	10	1.0	267	27	1880	0.46	0.56	4.6	14	41	867
Beef, ground	1 patty	163	18.8	9.1	0	11	175	2.8	66	301	20	0.08	0.17	4.5	0	9	367c
Ham	1 slice (1 oz.)	53	7.1	2.5	0	3	56	0	256	80		0.16	0.06	1.2			1771f
Hot dog	1	139	5.6	12.4	0.8	3	60	0.9	495	99		0.07	0.09	1.2			1994c
Bacon, crisp slices	2	86	3.8	7.8	0.5	2	34	0.5	153	35		0.08	0.05	0.8			126d
Cheese, processed	1 slice	100	6.3	8.1	0.5	188	208	0.2	307	22	330	0.1	0.11				653b
Egg, fried, large	1	99	6.3	7.9	0.1	28	102	1.1	155	64	650	0.05	0.14			28	968b
Margarine	1 t.	34	0	3.8	0	1	1		46	1	160						1317d
Potatoes, French fried	10	137	2.2	6.6	18.0	8	56	0.7	3	427		0.07	0.04	1.6	11	20	1789b
Lettuce	1 wedge (1/6 head)	9	0.6	0.1	2.0	14	15	0.4	6	123	230	0.04	0.04	0.2	4	30	1258g
Tomato	1	20	1.0	0.2	4.3	12	25	0.5	3	222	820	0.05	0.04	0.6	21	28	2282c
Coffee, instant	1 tsp.	1			0.3	1	3		1	26	0	0		0.2	0		799g
Soda, cola type	1 can	144	0		36.9												404a

[1]Household measure.
[2]Approximate values. All values are rounded to the nearest decimal point.
[3]Foods listed are available at fast-food restaurants and diners.
[4]Trace amount of this nutrient in the serving size indicated.
[5]Values given are from Agricultural Handbook No. 456. Nutritive value of American Foods. (USDA, Washington D.C.) except for total folacin values, which are from author's laboratory analysis of similar food items.

TABLE 9.3. FOOD AND NUTRITION BOARD, NATIONAL ACADEMY OF SCIENCES—NATIONAL RESEARCH COUNCIL RECOMMENDED DAILY DIETARY ALLOWANCES, REVISED 1974

Designed for the maintenance of good nutrition of practically all healthy people in the U.S.A.

	Age (years)	Weight (kg)	Weight (lbs)	Height (cm)	Height (in)	Energy (kcal)[a][b]	Protein (g)	Fat-Soluble Vitamins Vit. A Activity (RE)[c]	Vit. A (IU)	Vit. D (IU)	Vit. E Activity (IU)[e]	Water Soluble Vitamins Ascorbic Acid (mg)	Folacin (µg)[f]	Niacin (mg)[g]	Riboflavin (mg)	Thiamin (mg)	Vit. B6 (mg)	Vit. B12 (µg)	Minerals Calcium (mg)	Phosphorus (mg)	Iodine (µg)	Iron (mg)	Magnesium (mg)	Zinc (mg)
Infants	0.0–0.5	6	14	60	24	kg × 117	kg × 2.2	420[d]	1,400	400	4	35	50	5	0.4	0.3	0.3	0.3	360	240	35	10	60	3
	0.5–1.0	9	20	71	28	kg × 108	kg × 2.0	400	2,000	400	5	35	50	8	0.6	0.5	0.4	0.3	540	400	45	15	70	5
Children	1–3	13	28	86	34	1,300	23	400	2,000	400	7	40	100	9	0.8	0.7	0.6	1.0	800	800	60	15	150	10
	4–6	20	44	110	44	1,800	30	500	2,500	400	9	40	200	12	1.1	0.9	0.9	1.5	800	800	80	10	200	10
	7–10	30	66	135	54	2,400	36	700	3,300	400	10	40	300	16	1.2	1.2	1.2	2.0	800	800	110	10	250	10
Males	11–14	44	97	158	63	2,800	44	1,000	5,000	400	12	45	400	18	1.5	1.4	1.6	3.0	1,200	1,200	130	18	350	15
	15–18	61	134	172	69	3,000	54	1,000	5,000	400	15	45	400	20	1.8	1.5	2.0	3.0	1,200	1,200	150	18	400	15
	19–22	67	147	172	69	3,000	54	1,000	5,000	400	15	45	400	20	1.8	1.5	2.0	3.0	800	800	140	10	350	15
	23–50	70	154	172	69	2,700	56	1,000	5,000		15	45	400	18	1.6	1.4	2.0	3.0	800	800	130	10	350	15
	51+	70	154	172	69	2,400	56	1,000	5,000		15	45	400	16	1.5	1.2	2.0	3.0	800	800	110	10	350	15
Females	11–14	44	97	155	62	2,400	44	800	4,000	400	12	45	400	16	1.3	1.1	1.6	3.0	1,200	1,200	115	18	300	15
	15–18	54	119	162	65	2,100	48	800	4,000	400	12	45	400	14	1.4	1.1	2.0	3.0	1,200	1,200	115	18	300	15
	19–22	58	128	162	65	2,100	46	800	4,000	400	12	45	400	14	1.4	1.1	2.0	3.0	800	800	100	18	300	15
	23–50	58	128	162	65	2,000	46	800	4,000		12	45	400	13	1.2	1.0	2.0	3.0	800	800	100	18	300	15
	51+	58	128	162	65	1,800	46	800	4,000		12	45	400	12	1.1	1.0	2.0	3.0	800	800	80	10	300	15
Pregnant						+300	+30	1,000	5,000	400	15	60	800	+2	+0.3	+0.3	2.5	4.0	1,200	1,200	125	18+[h]	450	20
Lactating						+500	+20	1,200	6,000	400	15	80	600	+4	+0.5	+0.3	2.5	4.0	1,200	1,200	150	18	450	25

[a] The allowances are intended to provide for individual variations among most normal persons as they live in the United States under usual environmental stresses. Diets should be based on a variety of common foods in order to provide other nutrients for which human requirements have been less well defined. See text for more detailed discussion of allowances and of nutrients not tabulated. See Table I (p. 6) for weights and heights by individual year of age.

[b] Kilojoules (kJ) = 4.2 × kcal.

[c] Retinol equivalents.

[d] Assumed to be all as retinol in milk during the first six months of life. All subsequent intakes are assumed to be half as retinol and half as β-carotene when calculated from international units. As retinol equivalents, three fourths are as retinol and one fourth as β-carotene.

[e] Total vitamin E activity, estimated to be 80 percent as α-tocopherol and 20 percent other tocopherols. See text for variation in allowances.

[f] The folacin allowances refer to dietary sources as determined by *Lactobacillus casei* assay. Pure forms of folacin may be effective in doses less than one fourth of the Recommended Dietary Allowance.

[g] Although allowances are expressed as niacin, it is recognized that on the average 1 mg of niacin is derived from each 60 mg of dietary tryptophan.

[h] This increased requirement cannot be met by ordinary diets; therefore, the use of supplemental iron is recommended.

given in Table 9.2. For comparison of actual energy and nutrient intake from food with Recommended Dietary Allowances (RDA) reference can be made to Table 9.3. However, it must be understood that the RDA may be inadequate to meet the nutritional needs of an alcoholic. Total energy intake and total nutrient intake must include that obtained from alcoholic beverages.

MEDICAL HISTORY

The medical history can contribute to nutritional diagnosis, to comprehension of antecedent etiological factors, and to prediction of response to nutritional therapy.

The patient who has had single or recurrent episodes of illness which have resembled the presenting problem and which in the past has been clearly diagnosed as a nutritional disease, is more likely to receive a nutritional work-up and appropriate treatment.

In the alcoholic, etiological factors in the development of malnutrition may include not only inadequate food consumption, malabsorption, nutrient hyperexcretion, and impaired nutrient utilization, which are directly attributable to or alcohol-related, alcohol abuse diseases, but also trauma, infection, surgery, use of illicit drugs, and chronic intake of medications which interfere with nutritional status. History of previous and current illness can be obtained from the patient or patient's relatives, from his/her family physician, and/or from medical records. A very important figure which may best be derived from the history is the duration of alcohol abuse and the duration of alcohol related medical problems.

The treatment plan must be designed in accordance with past as well as present medical findings. For example, if a patient has had past episodes of liver failure, then dietary protein levels will be set to minimize risk of recurrence.

The functioning capacity of the patient should be determined by appropriate questioning both because this may offer clues on the nutritional diagnosis and assuredly because functional impairment may contribute to poor outcome of nutritional intervention. Included in the functional assessment are work status, e.g. the kind of job held, whether patient can work independently, ability and limitations for physical activity, absenteeism and health reasons, capacity to perform tasks in the home, especially tasks related to food purchase and meal preparation.

Symptoms are best recorded using a check list (Table 9.4). Symptoms in an alcoholic which suggest alcohol-related nutritional disease or

TABLE 9.4. CURRENT SYMPTOMS

Complaint	Yes	No	If yes, how often?			
			Constant	Daily	Weekly # times	Occasionally
Headache						
Insomnia						
Somnolence						
Excessive tiredness						
Nervousness						
Depression						
Blackouts						
Faintness						
Hangover						
Seizures						
Loss of memory						
Loss of appetite						
Loss of taste						
Sore tongue						
Bleeding gums						
Nausea						
Indigestion/flatulence						
Stomach pain						
Vomiting						
Diarrhea						
Muscle weakness						
Breathlessness on exertion						
Rash/dermatitis						

disease which can contribute to malnutrition are anorexia, early satiety, loss of taste, upper/lower abdominal pain, weight loss, muscle weakness, diarrhea, rash (generalized or localized to areas of trauma or U.V. exposure), breathlessness on exertion, and loss of memory.

Hillman (1974) indicates that symptoms can be divided into those which are suggestive of specific nutritional diseases and into those which are suggestive of conditioning disorders by which he means health complaints which influence either food intake or energy requirements.

Our experience has been that health complaints in the alcoholic are commonly multiple, that they are often hypochondriacal, and that the alcoholic, especially those with alcoholic brain syndromes, are extremely suggestible, so that confabulation obscures the significance of symptomatology. Indeed, whereas symptoms should be checked out in the physical examination, and may be due to alcohol-related disease productive of malnutrition, they are rarely related to nutritional disease.

PERSONAL FAMILY HISTORY

Demographic characteristics of patients should be ascertained. Basic information should include age, sex, education, marital status, household size and composition, living arrangements, occupation, income level and public assistance.

Access to food and alcohol should be determined and more particularly daily routine with respect to eating and drinking, working, using leisure time, social activities and sleep pattern.

PHYSICAL EXAMINATION

1. General

General appearance and behavior should be recorded including evidences of self-neglect, bodily habitus signs of inebriation, responsiveness or withdrawal, hypochondriasis, anxiety, depression, delusions, memory gaps, expression of hallucinations, and state of consciousness.

2. Anthropometric

Measurement of weight and height are required as well as measurements of mid upper arm circumference and triceps skinfold thickness. From these measurements, assessment of body fatness and lean body mass can be derived: the latter being reflected from calculation of arm muscle circumference.

Arm muscle circumference = arm circumference - [0.314 x triceps
       (cm)   (cm)   skinfold (mm)]

3. Clinical Nutrition Profile

Systems review should be aimed to achieve a comprehensive, objective definition of physical signs which may indicate nutritional deficiency or nutrient overload and/or alcoholic diseases contributing to or associated with nutritional disease. Abnormal physical findings other than obesity and cachexia cannot be accepted as diagnostic of nutritional disease unless the presumptive diagnosis, based on symptoms and signs, is supported by laboratory findings. In particular, lack of specificity of cutaneous and mucosal signs of avitaminoses including desquamation, localized or generalized dermatitis, purpura, angular stomatitis, glossitis, means that these signs can only be used to support a diagnosis of clinical malnutrition:

a) prospectively when tissue vitamin levels are depressed or when functional tests of vitamin status (WBC/RBC or platelets) indicate deficiency.

b) retrospectively when the abnormal signs clear in response to nutritional intervention. Preference for multivitamin therapy may preclude evaluation of the intervention test. Despite limitations which must be imposed on clinical nutritional diagnosis, physicians in working with alcoholics are more likely to miss clinical malnutrition than to misdiagnose individual or combined deficiency states. In order to assist clinical diagnosis of malnutrition, clinical features of nutritional deficiency diseases and of nutrient overload are summarized in Table 9.5.

LABORATORY INVESTIGATIONS

Laboratory tests can be divided into three groups:
1. Indicators of alcohol abuse.
2. Biochemical evidence of alcohol related disease.
3. Nutritional assessment.

In this category, laboratory procedures can be subdivided into:

a) tests which indicate inadequate nutrient intake or dietary imbalance:

b) tests which are diagnostic of specific nutrient deficiencies or overload. Biochemical assessment of nutritional status is commonly limited by the capabilities of hospital laboratories, but screening procedures for the most commonly encountered forms of malnutrition can usually be carried out.

TABLE 9.5.   CLINICAL SIGNS OF NUTRITIONAL DEFICIENCY AND OVERLOAD IN ALCOHOLICS

Nutrient Deficiency Overload	Skin	Subcut. Tissue	Muscle Skeleton	Mucous Membranes	Eyes	Blood	Intestinal	Heart	Peripheral	Brain	Genitalia	Syndrome
Food energy deficit		Loss of fat										Cachexia
Protein-energy deficit	Delayed wound healing	Edema	Wasting									Adult "Kwashiorkor"
Ascorbic acid deficiency	Delayed wound healing; purpura			Bleeding gums		Anemia						Scurvy
Niacin deficiency	Phototoxic dermatosis			Glossitis Stomatitis			Diarrhea Malabsorption			Confusional psychosis		Pellagra
Folacin deficiency				Glossitis Cheilitis		Anemia Macrocytic	Malabsorption			Organic brain syndrome		
Thiamin deficiency		Edema	Wasting					Congestive heart failure; wet beri-beri	Neuritis	Organic brain syndrome		Wernicke-Korsakoff syndrome beri-beri
Pyridoxine deficiency	Seborrhea Dermatitis					Anemia, Sideroblastic						
Riboflavin deficiency	Facial + scrotal dermatitis; angular stomatitis			Glossitis	Corneal vascularization				Neuritis			Ariboflavinosis
Vitamin B12 deficiency						Anemia, Macrocytic			Subacute combined degeneration			Post-gastrectomy anemia
Vitamin A deficiency					Night-blindness							
Vitamin D deficiency			Muscle weakness; bone softening + deformity									Osteomalacia
Vitamin K deficiency	Purpura						Blood loss					
Zinc deficiency	Acrodermatitis Erythroderma Delayed wound healing			Loss of taste								
Magnesium deficiency			Tetany					Cardiac arythmias		Tremor Seizures		
Potassium depletion			Muscle weakness									
Iron overload	Gray pigmentation; Loss of body hair									Testicular atrophy		Secondary hemochromatosis
Phosphate depletion			Myopathy									

1. Indicators of Alcohol Abuse

Biochemical and hematological aberrations have been proposed, as indicators of alcohol abuse. Rosalki *et al.* (1970) found that serum gamma glutamyl transpeptidase values were raised in approximately 75% of alcoholics. The suggestion that serum GGTP could be used as a useful screening test for alcoholism was made by Rollason *et al.* (1972). Subjects in the studies by Rollason and coworkers were males in a British health screening system who responded to a questionnaire about their drinking habits. Analysis of variance showed significant differences in GGTP values between drinking groups and greatest elevations found in those who reported that they drank six or more drinks per day. Since ethanol is an inducer of microsomal enzymes, and because hepatic as well as serum GGTP activities were found to be higher in ethanol fed rats than in pair fed controls, Teschke *et al.* (1977) suggested that changes in enzyme levels may be attributed to induction of hepatic microsomal GGTP.

Further studies of ethanol fed rats, carried out in Norway by Huseby *et al.* (1977) have produced information which challenges this hypothesis. The Norwegian investigators fed ethanol to rats as 34% of the calories of a liquid diet. Control rats were pair fed except that ethanol was replaced isocalorically by carbohydrate. After 1-7 weeks of ethanol feeding, experimental animals had higher GGTP activities in the plasma and liver than controls. Differences were not caused by elevation of GGTP activities in ethanol fed rats, but were due to a drop in values of control rats from zero time. The suggestion was made that the dietary carbohydrate may have suppressed GGTP activity in the controls.

Mezey (1978) supports this interpretation of findings, and comments that in order to test this hypothesis, it would be necessary to feed rats various levels of carbohydrate and then determine GGTP activities.

Whereas evidence to support the concept that GGTP is induced by ethanol is presently questioned, higher plasma levels in heavy drinkers than in abstainers may be explained, both on the basis of leakage of the enzyme from alcohol damaged hepatocytes, and on the basis of changes in carbohydrate intake or metabolism associated with alcohol abuse.

Whatever may be the reason for changes in GGTP with alcohol intake, the question arises whether this test offers promise in the clinic, hospital or community situation to screen for excessive alcohol consumption. Bircher and Preisig (1978), in reviewing earlier studies, comment on problems of interpreting GGTP values. They note that elevated values are met in cholestasis, in alcoholic liver disease, and in patients receiving phenobarbital or diphenylhydantoin (Whitfield *et al.,* 1972; Dragosics *et al.,* 1976).

An evaluation of biochemical and hematological markers of alcohol consumption has been carried out by Whitehead *et al.* (1978). They obtained blood samples from 2,034 British males aged 29-64 years, including 146 men whose alcohol consumption was known. Determinations were of GGTP, serum aspartate transaminase (AT), serum urate, serum triglyceride and mean corpuscular volume. As with GGTP, changes in these other blood parameters have been claimed to occur with alcohol abuse. Elevated GGTP or AT values, or both, were found in about one-fifth of the whole group, and in the subgroup, GGTP and AT rose with increasing alcohol intake. Correlation of serum urate with alcohol intake was found, and mean corpuscular volume also showed increases with alcohol consumption with drinking group differences being statistically significant between those who took 4 or more drinks per day and those who drank little or no alcohol.

Elevated serum triglyceride levels were related both to alcohol intake and to obesity. Subjects were all functioning well and had no obvious evidence of mental or physical disease. The authors consider that their data indicate that the "markers" are sensitive enough to pick out not only alcoholics but also social drinkers ("normal alcohol consumption").

We advocate retention of GGTP and mean corpuscular volume as markers of alcohol intake since differentiation of heavy drinkers is possible both in small group studies and in larger population surveys, and because repetition of tests will enable the investigator to find out whether there has been compliance with abstention achieved by alcoholics. These tests may also indicate alcohol abuse as a cause of malnutrition in those who do not admit to their drinking habits. GGTP values in alcoholics are usually > 30 mU/ml and a mean corpuscular volume > 93 cuμ in men and women without macrocytic anemia is indicative of alcohol abuse.

Plasma amino acid abnormalities may be indicative of alcoholism. Shaw and Lieber (1978) studied 56 alcoholics and 32 nonalcoholics with liver disease. Chronic alcohol consumption increased levels of branched chain amino acids. Advanced cirrhosis and also dietary protein deficiency depressed branched chain amino acid levels. The investigators indicated that in alcoholics plasma amino acids are affected by ethanol intake, dietary protein intake, and hepatic disease. Chronic alcohol consumption also increased alpha amino-n-butyric acid (AANB) levels but with dietary protein deficiency levels tended to be depressed. The authors suggest that the level of AANB in the plasma, expressed relative to leucine levels to correct for nutritional status, can be used as a biochemical marker to detect and assess the severity of alcoholism except in the circumstance that advanced cirrhosis is present.

2. Biochemical Evidence of Alcohol-Related Disease of the Intestine, Pancreas and Liver

a) **Intestine.**—Tests should include a panel which demonstrates dysfunctional capacity of the small intestine with respect to digestion and absorption. Choice of parameters and procedures should be on the basis of technical expertise as well as demonstration of abnormalities resulting from alcohol abuse.

Maldigestion can be identified by screening tests including determination of fecal fat and fecal nitrogen. If fecal nitrogen levels are elevated in stools collected for 3 days with a patient on a standard protein intake, the presence of protein losing enteropathy should be investigated by determining protein loss into the gastrointestinal tract by use of ^{51}Cr-albumin. Intestinal mucosal damage by ethanol can be identified by a lactose tolerance test and by measurement of disaccharidases and other brush border enzymes in jejunal biopsy specimens.

Appropriate screening tests for malabsorption include the D-xylose absorption test and plasma carotene levels. Proximal intestinal malabsorption can be studied by thiamin, and folacin absorption tests. Distal intestinal malabsorption can be identified by the Schilling test.

In the alcoholic, differentiation of maldigestion from malabsorption is by the D-xylose test which may be normal in cases of maldigestion. A critical review of tests of intestinal absorption has been published by Russell and Lee (1978). (See also van de Kamer *et al.*, 1949; Wilson and Dietschy, 1971; Waldmann, 1966; Finlay *et al.*, 1964; Wenger *et al.*, 1957; Tomasulo, 1958; Lamar *et al.*, 1965.)

b) **Pancreas.**—Abnormalities of pancreatic function follow regular heavy alcohol consumption. It is known, from the work of Sarles (1975) and Sarles *et al.* (1965) that chronic calcifying pancreatitis is the common pancreatic disease of alcoholics, though these same pancreatic changes can be found in protein deficiency. The illness is characterized by exacerbations and remissions. Acute pancreatitis is liable to supervene, particularly in the earlier phases of the illness. Laboratory tests may be divided into serum enzyme measurements, used in the diagnosis of acute pancreatitis, studies of pancreatic secretory capacity which may validate the clinical diagnosis of chronic pancreatitis, and tests of digestive capacity which determine pancreatic exocrine function. Serum enzyme levels include serum amylase and serum lipase. Diagnostic procedures which are applied in suspected chronic pancreatitis are a) Trypsin output after a standard liquid meal* and b) Bicarbonate concentration of duodenal aspirates after secretion stimulation. Output of trypsin and lipase in response to cholecystokinin-pancreozymin (CCK-PZ) decrease with time in alcoholics.

Evaluation of pancreatic secretory function tests is given by Wormsley (1978). Discussion of effects of chronic alcoholism on pancreatic function and functional tests is reviewed by Mowat and Brunt (1978). According to Harvey et al. (1973), CCK-PZ levels are higher in patients with alcoholic pancreatic disease of long duration.

Steatorrhea occurs late in the course of chronic alcoholic pancreatitis, and is associated with reduced lipase outputs in response to CCK-PZ. Elevated fecal nitrogen (creatorrhea) occurs when stimulated trypsin levels fall below 10% of normal maximal output (DiMagno et al., 1975).

c) Liver.—Serum glutamic oxaloacetic (SGOT) and serum glutamic pyruvic transaminase (SGPT) levels have withstood the test of 20 years' use as liver function tests, which indicate damage to the hepatocyte. While numerous drugs cause liver injury, ethanol is the commonest liver poison and therefore elevation of serum levels of these transaminases caused by leakage of these enzymes from the hepatocytes is commonly due to alcohol abuse. (The assumption is made that infectious hepatitis can be excluded.)

According to Harinasuta et al. (1967), in alcoholic hepatitis or steatonecrosis, SGOT values are usually less than 250 units and SGPT values less than 150 units. In alcoholic hepatitis and in cirrhosis, the SGOT:SGPT ratio is greater than 1.0. In alcoholic hepatitis, serum bilirubin, alkaline phosphatase and lactic dehydrogenase (LDH) levels are also increased. Hypoprothrombinemia is frequently present with the greater prolongation of prothrombin time being present in patients with the most severe alcoholic hepatitis. Hyperammonemia occurs with incipient hepatic encephalopathy in alcoholic hepatitis and cirrhosis. Fatty liver (steatosis), alcoholic hepatitis, and cirrhosis can only be diagnosed conclusively by examination of liver biopsies.

Biochemical differentiation of alcoholic hepatitis from cirrhosis is by normal LDH values in cirrhosis, by hypoalbuminemia and hyperglobulinemia in cirrhosis, and by higher bilirubin (conjugated) in hepatitis. Bilirubinuria may occur in alcoholic hepatitis (Sherlock, 1955).

*The Lundh test consists in administration of a test meal containing 5% protein, 6% fat and 15% carbohydrate and collection of pancreatic secretion for determination of tryptic activity using a specific substrate (N-1-benzoyl-1-arginine-ethylester). Arvanitakis and Cooke (1978) comment on the simplicity of the test and its usefulness in the diagnosis of chronic pancreatitis.

Increased serum iron levels occur in cirrhosis and in iron overload (secondary hemochromatosis) both serum iron and serum ferritin levels may be raised (Prieto *et al.,* 1975). Total iron binding capacity (TIBC) of the serum is also saturated in hemochromatosis. Diagnosis of iron overload disease in alcoholics is by these tests showing excess iron in the circulation, by the positive Prussian blue test on the skin, and by histochemical demonstration of iron deposition in liver biopsy samples (Powell, 1975).

3. Biochemical Assessment of Nutritional Status.—

Limitations of expertise, methodology and facilities, as well as the constraints of time, require that tests for the biochemical determination of the nutritional status of alcoholics be selected according to guidelines derived from knowledge of magnitude of risk of particular nutritional disorders and the circumstances which condition occurrence. Since dietary information may be inaccurate, there is justification for choice of tests which reflect recent intake as well as tests which denote real abnormalities in the nutritional condition of the patient.

4. Use and Abuse of Biochemical Measures to Assess Nutrient Intake

a) **Protein.**—Urinary urea-creatinine ratio has been proposed as a measure of dietary protein intake. Measurement of urinary urea nitrogen and urinary creatinine in 24 hr. urine samples or random urine samples allows calculation of the urea creatinine ratio from the following formula:

$$\text{urea-creatinine ratio} = \frac{\text{mg urea nitrogen/ml urine}}{\text{mg creatinine/ml urine}}$$

Validity of urea nitrogen/creatinine ratios as a measure of protein intake are discussed by Simmons (1972). Whether or not urine samples are obtained in the fasting or feasted state affects urinary urea nitrogen values with more being excreted after a meal. Hence, random urine samples cannot be used. Urinary urea nitrogen levels vary with diuresis, maximum values occurring with high urine flow. Fluid intake and diuretic drugs will influence findings, and unless these factors can be controlled, use of urinary urea nitrogen values as a measure of protein intake will be misleading (Arroyave, 1962).

It has been questioned whether urea nitrogen/creatinine ratio is an indicator of the level of recent protein intake or also of dietary protein quality. Simmons was of the opinion that the ratio reflects dietary protein quantity and quality.

According to Blackburn et al. (1977), measurement of 24 hour urinary urea nitrogen can be used to evaluate the degree of hypermetabolism or tissue breakdown in hospitalized patients. The assumption is that in the catabolic state urinary urea nitrogen excretion will no longer be related to protein intake but rather to the rate and severity of tissue breakdown.

Alcohol per se has a complex effect on urinary urea nitrogen loss, such that when given as a supplemental energy source, it can be nitrogen sparing and when given as an isocaloric substitute for carbohydrate in the diet, urea nitrogen excretion may be increased. The complexities in evaluating the meaning of urinary urea nitrogen values strongly detract from the usefulness of these measurements more particularly in alcoholics as a determinant of protein intake (Shar and Lieber, 1977; Klatskin, 1961; Rodrigo et al., 1971).

b) Vitamins.

(1) Ascorbic acid.—It has been established that, over a limited range of values, plasma levels of ascorbic acid show a linear relationship to intake of vitamin C. Concentration of plasma ascorbic acid decreases rapidly with dietary deprivation. Above a certain level of intake plasma levels plateau although with sudden very high intake levels in the plasma may increase briefly. Low plasma levels of ascorbic acid do imply deficient intake but are not diagnostic of scurvy. With a very low or zero intake of the vitamin, excretion of ascorbic acid in the urine ceases. Plasma ascorbic acid levels are lower in heavy smokers and therefore because alcoholics are commonly in this smoking category, a finding of low plasma levels may not necessarily imply low dietary intake of vitamin C. Contraceptive steroids also lead to depression of plasma ascorbic acid levels and therefore in female alcoholics, it is important to ascertain whether or not they are on the Pill (Sauberlich, 1975; Rivers and Devine, 1972).

(2) Riboflavin.—It has been established that relationships exist between riboflavin intake and urinary riboflavin excretion. Clinical signs of riboflavin deficiency develop in men on an intake of 0.55 mg/day and at this level of intake urinary riboflavin is in the range of 20-30 μg/g creatinine. Urinary excretion of riboflavin slowly increases with intake until at a level of 1.3 - 1.6 mg/day urinary excretion of riboflavin suddenly increases, indicating saturation of the renal tubular reabsorption mechanism. A similar pattern of riboflavin excretion in relation to intake is seen in women. Whereas riboflavin excretion is definitely related to

recent intake of the vitamin, hyperexcretion occurs with fasting, heavy exercise, injury, burns, elevated body temperature, and ingestion of borate. In the alcoholic these causes of riboflavinuria may pertain. On the other hand, low excretion of riboflavin in the alcoholic may be due to malabsorption (Horwitt et al., 1950; Jusko and Levy, 1975; Pinto et al., 1978).

(3) Thiamin.—Urinary excretion of thiamin, best measured as µg thiamine/g creatinine in 24-hr urine samples, is related to intake such that with reduced intake urinary thiamin decreases to a set level such that with further dietary depletion, there is no further lowering of urinary values for the vitamin. Low urinary levels of thiamin occur in beri-beri and other thiamin deficiency syndromes. However, in alcoholics, low urinary thiamin levels may also be due to malabsorption of the vitamin (Sauberlich et al., 1974; Thompson et al., 1970).

(4) Folacin.—Plasma folacin levels are related in persons who are not imbibing alcohol to total folacin intake. However, consumption of alcohol causes a precipitous fall in plasma folacin. Other factors, unrelated to diet, which cause lowering of plasma folacin are intake of certain drugs including contraceptive steroids, diphenylhydantoin and phenobarbital. Malabsorption due to toxic effects of ethanol on the intestinal mucosa, to drugs such as salicylazosulfapyridine, to intestinal diseases such as gluten-sensitive enteropathy and due to late effects of partial gastrectomy, impairs folacin absorption and, hence, is associated with low plasma folacin levels. In the alcoholic, use of plasma folacin as an indicator of folacin intake is unreliable (Roe and Liebman, 1977; Eichner and Hillman, 1973; Halsted et al., 1971; Jensen and Olesen, 1970; Spray, 1968; Franklin and Rosenberg, 1973; Mahmud et al., 1974; Bernstein et al., 1970).

(5) Vitamin B_6.—The urinary excretion of vitamin B_6 is related to the level of recent intake of the vitamin. Measurement is rarely of use in alcoholics because alcohol-induced vitamin B_6 deficiency is due to inhibition of pyridoxal kinase and diminished synthesis of pyridoxal phosphate by ethanol (Hines, 1975).

(6) Vitamin A.—Plasma levels of carotene and retinol are related to dietary levels of these nutrients but do not accurately reflect recent intake of vitamin A sources. Further, in the alcoholic, low levels of plasma carotene may be associated with malabsorption and low levels of plasma retinol may denote concurrent protein deficiency or zinc deficiency. It is not recommended that plasma levels of either carotene or retinol be accepted as measures of vitamin A intake in alcohol abusers (Patwardhan, 1969; Sauberlich et al., 1974; Cassidy et al., 1978).

4. Diagnostic Tests for Specific Nutrient Deficiencies and Overload in Alcoholics

a) Protein.—*Visceral protein status,* which implies the body's capacity for protein synthesis, and particularly hepatic protein synthesis, can most easily be investigated by measuring *serum albumin* and *serum transferrin.* For nutritional screening purposes, the serum transferrin value can be derived from estimations of total iron binding capacity:

$$\text{Serum transferrin} = (0.8 \times \text{TIBC}) -43$$

Peripheral protein status (lean body mass or change in lean body mass) can be estimated from comparisons of the creatinine excretion of the patient to that of an "ideal" or standard person of the same height. In practice, the *creatinine height index* is computed from the 24-hour urinary excretion of creatinine of the patient and use of a table of "ideal" urinary creatinine values as follows:

$$\text{Creatinine height index (CHI)} = \frac{\text{Actual urinary creatinine} \times 100}{\text{Ideal urinary creatinine}}$$

(Gaber *et al.,* 1971; Whitehead *et al.,* 1971; Arroyave and Wilson, 1961; Bistrian *et al.,* 1975).

Hair root diameter measurement has been proposed by Bregar *et al.* (1978) as a measure of the protein status of non-hospitalized alcoholics. Mean hair diameters of 84 alcoholics averaged 0.086 ± 0.037 mm as compared with values of 0.100 ± 0.025 mm for non-alcoholic controls. The percent of telogen (non-growing) and atrophied anagen (growing) hair also differed in alcoholics. The specificity of hair measurements as an index of protein status in alcoholics needs further investigation, particularly since an abnormal distribution of telogen hairs and atrophied anagen hairs may occur with fasting which is not uncommon during alcoholic sprees. Further the number of measurements which are required for such an assessment limit usefulness of the method in a clinical setting.

b) Zinc and Vitamin A.—Zinc metabolism is altered in alcoholic cirrhosis. Hyperzincuria is associated with alcohol abuse and alcoholic liver disease. Measurement of serum and urinary zinc is recommended in the assessment of the nutrition of alcoholics with biochemical and histological evidence of liver disease. Special indications for determinations of zinc status are:

(1) Zinc clearance to monitor the progress of alcoholic liver disease. Increased renal clearance of zinc denotes deterioration in the hepatic condition and conversely decreased renal clearance of zinc indicates improvement.

(2) Serum zinc to ascertain the zinc nutrition of alcoholics prior to surgery when interruption in food intake as well as the catabolic effects of surgery may precipitate clinical zinc deficiency.

(3) Serum zinc in patients who have one or more of the following clinical signs: loss of taste, delayed wound healing, generalized scaling dermatosis or pyoderma which may be indicative of zinc deficiency.

(4) Serum zinc and plasma retinol in patients who either complain of difficulty in seeing at night or who have had accidents at night due to visual problems. Vitamin A deficiency may be secondary to zinc deficiency in alcoholics.

Plasma retinol as well as plasma retinol binding protein (RBP) and prealbumin, a third component of the RBP-retinol complex, have been found to be significantly depressed in patients with liver disease including those with cirrhosis. Zinc deficiency with low serum zinc levels as well as vitamin A deficiency with depressed plasma retinol and RBP levels are found in alcoholics with cirrhosis who may have nightblindness (Allen *et al.*, 1975; Davies *et al.*, 1968; Halsted and Smith, 1974; Smith *et al.*, 1973; Cassidy *et al.*, 1978).

c) **Thiamin.**—Erythrocyte transketolase determinations can be used to indicate a functional deficiency of thiamin. Transketolase is a thiamin-pyrophosphate dependent enzyme in the pentose phosphate pathway which functions in the interconversion of pentoses. Thiamin deficiency in the alcoholic may be due to inadequate intake or malabsorption, due possibly to an inability of the alcoholic to dephosphorylate thiamin in the intestine, which is necessary to absorption of the vitamin. Alcoholics who develop the Wernicke-Korsakoff syndrome may have a genetic abnormality in their transketolase which may make them thiamin-dependent. It has been suggested that with thiamin depletion alcoholics having the abnormal transketolase apoenzyme develop the Wernicke-Korsakoff syndrome,whreas other alcoholics, whosee transketolase is normal, do not run this risk. Patients with this disease show reduced ereythrocyte transketolase activity which, however, returns toward normal values after parenteral injection of thiamin (Dreyfus, 1962; Brin, 1962; Baker *et al.*, 1975; Blass and Gibson, 1977).

d) **Riboflavin.**—Riboflavin status can be assessed by erythrocyte glutathione reductase (EGR) assay. The EGR enzyme which catalyses reduction of oxidized glutathione has flavin (FAD) as cofactor. Presently this is the best available method for determination of riboflavin status, although values are influenced by recent riboflavin intake and therefore may not reflect tissue flavin storage. The sensitivity of the test for the determination of riboflavin status of alcoholics has been affirmed by Rosenthal et al. (1973) and Tillotson and Baker (1972).

e) **Folacin, Vitamin B$_{12}$, Vitamin B$_6$, and Iron.**—Alcohol-related diseases which may be related to deficiencies in B vitamin nutriture are anemias and iron overload. Evidence suggests that with chronic alcohol abuse hemopoiesis is disturbed such that there are maturational defects in precursur cells and defects in heme synthesis. The hematological effects of alcohol are due to direct effects of alcohol and to alcohol-induced nutritional defects which lead to both megaloblastic and sideroblastic anemias, which may be co-existent. Complex and multiple effects of alcohol abuse on hemopoiesis may be associated with combined folacin, vitamin B$_{12}$ and vitamin B$_6$ deficiencies. Biochemical evaluations of the tissue stores of these vitamins as well as functional impairment requires that the investigator understands that conventional tests may yield misleading information.

The following conditions require combined studies of folacin, vitamin B$_{12}$, vitamin B$_6$ and iron status.

(1) macrocytosis without anemia.
(2) megaloblastic anemia with or without neurological signs indicative of vitamin B$_{12}$ deficiency.
(3) combined sideroblastic and megaloblastic anemia.
(4) post-gastrectomy anemia.
(5) anemia associated with GI blood loss.
(6) hemolytic anemia.
(7) bone marrow evidence of iron overload (hemosiderosis).
(8) failure in response of alcoholics with anemia to single hematinics.

NUTRITIONAL PROFILE NEEDED

A nutritional profile which should be obtained in these conditions is as follows:

a) **Folacin:** Determination of plasma + erythrocyte folacin and FIGLU test. Herbert et al. (1973) and Herbert and Tisman (1975) also recommended the dU suppression test. Even if biochemical evidence is obtained of folacin deficiency including erythrocyte folacin levels in the deficient range, it cannot be assumed that this is an isolated deficiency except by therapeutic trial of folic acid.

b) Vitamin B$_{12}$: In the alcoholic, vitamin B$_{12}$ hepatic stores may be depleted due to low intake, malabsorption or inadequate storage potential of the cirrhotic liver. Serum levels of vitamin B$_{12}$ may not reflect B$_{12}$ stores in patients with alcoholic cirrhosis, and it has been demonstrated that alcoholics with normal or elevated serum B$_{12}$ levels and megaloblastosis may respond to vitamin B$_{12}$ administration. It is recommended that serum vitamin B$_{12}$ levels be measured but that in addition urinary methyl malonic acid (MMA) be determined. Elevated excretion of MMA is characteristic of vitamin B$_{12}$ deficiency (Kahn *et al.*, 1965; Skeggs, 1963; Raven *et al.*, 1971).

c) Vitamin B$_6$: Following the experience of Hines (1975), it is recommended that assessment of vitamin B$_6$ status in alcoholics should include determinations of serum and whole blood pyridoxal phosphate. Values for both these parameters are significantly reduced in alcoholics, indicating defective synthesis of the coenzyme form of the vitamin.

d) Iron: When precursor red cells in bone marrow smears are found to contain excess iron, as determined by histochemical staining, serum iron and serum ferritin levels should be measured. Hyperferremia occurs in association with sideroblastosis. Both the hyperferremia and the sideroblastosis are reversed by administration of pyridoxal phosphate. However, when hemochromatosis occurs in alcoholics, hyperferremia is not altered by pyridoxal phosphate (Jacobs and Worwood, 1975).

Megaloblastic anemia in alcoholics is most commonly due to folacin deficiency. After gastrointestinal blood loss, iron deficiency anemia will develop with hyperferremia but in addition megaloblastic anemia, due to folacin deficiency, may ensue because of excessive demands for this nutrient for the maturation of precursor red cells. Similarly, in hemolytic anemias of alcoholics with liver disease, folacin stores may be reduced and secondary folacin deficient megaloblastic anemia may occur, especially in alcoholics on low folacin intakes. Both with GI blood loss and in the presence of hemolytic anemia, erythrocyte folacin levels may be in the deficient range. Vitamin B$_{12}$ deficiency may occur in alcoholics who have had a partial gastrectomy as well as in those with cirrhosis.

Due to the interactive effects of alcohol and those B vitamins (that is, folacin, vitamin B$_{12}$ and vitamin B$_6$) in causing hematological disorders and the possible influence of ethanol ingestion on test results, it is recommended that laboratory studies be performed during or immediately following an alcoholic spree and that tests be repeated after a two week period of abstinence (Chanarin, 1969).

e) Niacin: Determination of niacin status is recommended a) when the patient's diet has been pellagrogenic; b) when there are cutaneous GI and neurological signs of chronic pellagra; c) when the patient has combined glossitis, stomatitis, indigestion, diarrhea, indicative of acute pellagra; and d) in patients with carcinoid tumors.

Sauberlich *et al.* (1974) advocates use of procedures for estimating N^1-methylnicotinamide excretion and the ratio of the urinary niacin metabolites 2-pyridone and N^1-methylnicotinamide.

f) Ascorbic Acid: Ascorbic acid status should be assessed in alcoholics who have subsisted on a scorbutic diet, in those with signs suggestive of scurvy as well as in alcoholics who show drug intolerance. Vitamin C is required in drug metabolism. The optimal method for assessing tissue stores is by measurement of leukocyte ascorbate. It is, however, easier to perform ascorbic acid saturation tests which will establish whether or not a vitamin deficiency is present (Beattie and Sherlock, 1976; Lowry *et al.,* 1946).

MINERAL MACRONUTRIENTS: SODIUM, POTASSIUM AND MAGNESIUM

Serum electrolyte determinations must be performed:

1) on all alcoholics admitted to hospital following prolonged alcoholic debauch whether hospitalization is for detoxication, treatment of injury or infection.

2) in alcoholics requiring surgery or after surgery.

3) in patients with alcoholic heart disease and undiagnosed cardiac arythmias.

4) in alcoholics having cirrhosis with or without ascites and after paracentesis.

5) in alcoholics receiving diuretics.

Hypokalemia is common in alcoholics and may result from potassium losses associated with prolonged vomiting, diarrhea, and oral diuretics.

Hyponatremia in alcoholics with cirrhosis is most likely to follow diuretic therapy. Usually it is symptomless but as noted by Sherlock (1963), may be the herald of hepatic encephalopathy. With oral diuretic therapy, combined hyponatremia and hypokalemia occurs. Hypokalemia is corrected by stopping the diuretic and giving a high potassium diet (potassium chloride may be given in severe depletion). Hyponatremia should not be treated by salt feeding, but will respond to discontinuation of the causal diuretic and administration of mannitol.

Paracentesis can cause sodium depletion especially if the alcoholic has been on a sodium-restricted diet. Cramps, weakness and hypotension in these circumstances will suggest hyponatremia (Rawsey *et al.*, 1953).

Serum magnesium determination is indicated in patients during alcohol detoxication, especially in those exhibiting signs of withdrawal syndromes. Other indications are thiamin deficiency in which signs are potentiated by magnesium lack. Analysis is by atomic absorption spectrometry (Willis, 1965).

Table 9.6 lists biochemical tests used in screening alcoholics with respect to their nutritional status. It also shows normal values and indicates values associated with nutritional deficiencies or overload.

TABLE 9.6.　BIOCHEMICAL ASSESSMENT OF NUTRITIONAL STATUS IN ALCOHOLICS

Nutrient Evaluation	Test	Unit	Acceptable[a] Values	Indicates Deficiency	Indicates Overload	Remarks and Intermediate Values
Protein	Serum albumin	g/100 ml	⩾3.5	<2.8		Low values 2.8-3.4
Thiamin	Erythrocyte transketolase	%TPP stimulation	0-15	>20		TPP=thiamin pyrophosphate. Medium risk 16-20
Riboflavin	Erythrocyte glutathione reductase	activity coefficients	<1.2	>1.4		Medium risk 1.2-1.4
Folacin	Plasma folacin	ng/ml	>6.0	<3.0		Low values 3.0-5.9
	Erythrocyte folacin	ng/ml	>160	<140		Low values 140-159
Niacin	N'-methylnicotinamide excretion	mg/g creatinine	1.60-4.29	<0.50		Low values 0.5-1.59
Pyridoxine (Vitamin B₆)	Serum pyridoxal (PLP) phosphate	ng/ml	30-60	<20		Low values 20-29
	Whole blood PLP	ng/ml	⩾115	<80		Low values 80-114
Vitamin B₁₂	Serum vitamin B₁₂	pg/ml	>200	<150		Low values 150-200
Vitamin C	Serum ascorbic acid	mg/100 ml	⩾0.30	<0.20		Low values 0.20-0.29
Vitamin A	Plasma retinol	μg/100 ml	20-70	<10	>80	Low values 10-19
Vitamin D	caxp product	mg%	⩾40	<30		Low values 30-39
Iron	Serum iron	μg/100 ml	60-169	<50	>170	
	Transferrin saturation [b]	%	20-50	<15		
	Serum ferritin	μg/ml	12-180	<12	c	
Zinc	Serum zinc	μg/dl	75-140	<60		
Magnesium	Serum magnesium	mEq/1	1.3-2.0	<1.3		
Potassium	Serum potassium	mEq/1	4.0-5.0	<4.0		
Sodium	Serum sodium	mEq/1	135-145	<135		

[a] Values are taken from the following sources: Sauberlich et al., 1974; Wands et al., 1976; Hines, 1975.

[b] Percent transferrin saturation $= \left(\dfrac{\text{serum iron in } \mu g/100 \text{ ml}}{\text{TIBC in } \mu g/100 \text{ ml}} \right) \times 100$

[c] Values above upper limits are not precise indicators of overload.

SELECTED REFERENCES

Allen, J.G., Fell, G.S. and Russell, R.I. 1975. Urinary zinc in hepatic cirrhosis. Scott. Med. J. 20: 109-111.

Arroyave, G. 1962. The estimation of relative nutrient intake and nutritional status by biochemical methods: Problems. Amer. J. Clin. Nutr. 11: 447-461.

Arroyave, G. and Wilson, D. 1961. Urinary excretion of creatinine of children under different nutritional conditions. Amer. J. Clin. Nutr. 9: 170-175.

Arvanitakis, C. and Cooke, A.R. 1978. Diagnostic tests of exocrine pancreatic function and disease. Gastroenterology 74: 932-948.

Baker, H., Frank, O., Zetterman, R.K., Rajan, K.S., ten Hove, W. and Leevy, C.M. 1975. Inability of chronic alcoholics with liver disease to use food as a source of folates, thiamin and vitamin B6. Amer. J. Clin. Nutr. 28: 1377-1380.

Beattie, A.D. and Sherlock, S. 1976. Ascorbic acid deficiency in liver disease. Gut 17: 571-575.

Bernstein, L.H., Gutstein, S., Werner, S. and Efron, G. 1970. The absorption and malabsorption of folic acid and its polyglutamates. Amer. J. Med. 48: 570-579.

Bircher, J. and Preisig, R. 1978. Excretory liver function tests. Clin. Gastroenterol. 7, #2, 517-528.

Bistrian, B.R., Blackburn, G.L., Sherman, M. et al. 1975. Therapeutic index of nutritional depletion in hospitalized patients. Surg. Gynecol. Obstet. 141: 512-516.

Blackburn, G.L., Bistrian,B.R., Maini, B.S., Schlamm, H.T. and Smith, M.F. 1977. Nutritional and metabolic assessment of the hospitalized patient. J. Parenteral and Enteral Nutr. 1: 11-22.

Blass, J.P. and Gibson, G.E. 1977. Abnormality of a thiamine-requiring enzyme in patients with Wernicke-Korsakoff syndrome. New Eng. J. Med. 297: 1367-1370.

Bregar, R.R., Gordon, M. and Whitney, E.N. 1978. Hair root diameter measurements as an indicator of protein deficiency in non-hospitalized alcoholics. Amer. J. Clin. Nutr. 31: 230-236.

Brin, M. 1962. Erythrocyte transketolase in early thiamine deficiency. Ann. N.Y. Acad. Sci. 98: 528-541.

Burke, B.S. 1947. The dietary history as a tool in research. J. Am. Diet. Assoc. 23: 1041-1046.

Cassidy, W.A., Brown, E.D. and Cecil Smith, J. Jr. 1978. Alterations in zinc and vitamin A metabolism in alcoholic liver disease: A review. In Zinc and Copper in Clinical Medicine, Eds. Michael Hambridge, K. and Nichols, B.L. Jr. New York, London: SP Medical and Scientific Books. pp. 59-79.

Chanarin, I. 1969. The Megaloblastic Anemias. Oxford and Edinburgh: Blackwell Scientific Publ. pp. 389-391.

Chanarin, I., Anderson, B.B. and Mollin, D.L. 1958. The absorption of folic acid. Brit. J. Haemat. 4: 156-166.

Davies, I.J.T., Musa, M. and Dormandy, T.L. 1968. Measurements of plasma zinc. J. Clin. Path. 21: 359-365.

DiMagno, E.P., Malagelada, J.R. and Go. V.L.W. 1975. Relationship between alcoholism and pancreatic insufficiency. Ann. N.Y. Acad. Sci. 252: 200-207.

Dragosics, B., Ferenci, P., Pesendorfer, F. and Wewalka, F.G. 1976. Gamma-glutamyl transpeptidase (GGTP): Its relationship to other enzymes for diagnosis of liver disease. In *Progress in Liver Disease*, Eds. Popper, H. and Schaffner, F. New York: Grune and Stratton. pp. 436-449.

Dreyfus, P.M. 1962. Clinical application of blood transketolase determinations. New Eng. J. Med. 267: 596-598.

Eagles, J.A. and Longman, D. 1963. Reliability of alcoholics reports of food intake. J. Amer. Dietet. Assoc. 42: 136-139.

Eichner, E.R. and Hillman, R.S. 1973. Effect of alcohol on serum folate level. J. Clin. Invest. 52: 584-591.

Finlay, J.M., Hogarth, J., and Wightman, R.J. 1964. A clinical evaluation of the D-xylose tolerance test. Ann. Intern. Med. 61: 411-422.

Franklin, J. and Rosenberg, I.H. 1973. Impaired folic acid absorption in inflammatory bowel disease: Effects of salicylazosulfapyridine (Azulfidine). Gastroenterology 64: 517-525.

Gabr, M. El-Hawary, M.F., and El-Dali, M. 1971. Serum transferrin in kwashiorkor. J. Trop. Med. Hyg. 74: 216-221.

Halsted, C.H., Robles, E.A. and Mezey, E. 1971. Decreased jejunal uptake of labelled folic acid (^{3}H-PGA) in alcoholic patients: roles of alcohol and nutrition. New Eng. J. Med. 285: 701-706.

Halsted, J.A. and Smith, J.C. Jr. 1974. Night blindness and chronic liver disease. Gastroenterology 67: 193-194.

Harinasuta, U., Chomet, B., Ishak, K. and Zimmerman, H.J. 1967. Steatonecrosis-Mallory body type. Medicine 46: 141-162.

Harvey, R.F., Dowsett, L., Hartog, M. and Read, A.E. 1973. A radioimmunoassay for cholecystokinin pancreozymin. Lancet 2: 826-827.

Herbert, V. and Tisman, G. 1975. Hematologic effects of alcohol. Ann. N.Y. Acad. Sci. 252: 307-315.

Herbert, V., Tisman, G., Go, L.T. and Brenner, L. 1973. The dU-suppression test using ^{125}IUdR to define biochemical megaloblastosis. Brit. J. Haemat. 24: 713-723.

Hillman, R.W. 1974. Alcoholism and malnutrition. In *The Biology of Alcoholism*, Vol. 3, Clinical Pathology. Eds. Kissin, B. and Begleiter, H. New York: Plenum Press. pp. 513-586.

Hines, J.D. 1975. Hematologic abnormalities involving vitamin B6 and folate metabolism in alcoholic subjects. Ann. N.Y. Acad. Sci. 252: 316-327.

Horwitt, M.K., Harvey, C.C., Hills, O.W. and Liebert, E. 1950. Correlation of urinary excretion of riboflavin with dietary intake and symptoms of aribo-flavinosis. J. Nutr. 41: 247-264.

Jacobs, A. and Worwood, M. 1975. The biochemistry of ferritin and its clini-cal implications. In *Progress in Hematology*, Vol. IX. Ed. Brown, E.B. New York, San Francisco, London: Grune and Stratton. pp. 1-24.

Jensen, O.N. and Oleson, O.V. 1970. Subnormal serum folate due to anticon-vulsive therapy: a double-blind study of the effect of folic acid treatment in patients with drug-induced subnormal serum folates. Arch. Neurol. 22: 181-182.

Jusko, W.J. and Levy, G. 1975. Absorption, protein binding and elimination of riboflavin. In *Riboflavin*. Ed. Rivlin, R.S. New York and London: Ple-num Press. pp. 99-152.

Kahn, S.B., Williams, W.J., Barness, L.A., Young, D., Shafer, B., Vivacqua, R.J. and Beaupre, E.M. 1965. Methylmalonic acid excretion: A sensitive indica-tor of vitamin B12 deficiency in man. J. Lab. Clin. Med. 66: 75-83.

Klatskin, G. 1961. The effect of ethyl alcohol on nitrogen excretion in the rat (Abst.). Yale J. Biol. Med. 34: 124.

Lamar, C., McCracken, B.H., Miller, O.N. and Goldsmith, G.A. 1965. Exper-iences with the Schilling test as a diagnostic tool. Amer. J. Clin. Nutr. 16: 402-411.

Lowry, O.H., Bessey, O.A., Brock, M.J. and Lopez, J.A. 1946. The interrela-tionship of dietary, serum, white blood cell and total body ascorbic acid. J. Biol. Chem. 166: 111-119.

Mahmud, K., Kaplan, M.E., Ripley, D., Swaim, M.A. and Doscherhobnen, A. 1974. The importance of red cell B12 and folate levels after partial gastrec-tomy. Amer. J. Clin. Nutr. 27: 51-54.

Mezey, E. 1978. Alcohol consumption and α-glutamyl transferase activity. Gastroenterology 74: 632-633.

Morland, J., Huseby, N.E., Sjoblom, M. and Stromme, J.H. 1977. Does chronic alcohol consumption really induce hepatic microsomal gamma-glutamyl transferase activity? Biochem. Biophys. Res. Commun. 77: 1060-1066.

Mowat, N.A.G. and Brunk, P.W. 1976. Alcohol and the gastrointestinal tract. In *Recent Advances in Gastroenterology*. Ed. Bouchier, I.A.D. Edinburgh, London, New York: Churchill, Livingstone.

Patwardhan, V.N. 1969. Hypovitaminosis A and epidemiology of xeroph-thalmia. Amer. J. Clin. Nutr. 22: 1106-1118.

Pinto, J., Huang, Y.P., McConnell, R.J. and Rivlin, R.S. 1978. Increased urinary riboflavin excretion resulting from boric acid ingestion. J. Lab. Clin. Med. 92: 126-134.

Powell, L.W. 1975. The role of alcoholism in hepatic iron storage disease. Ann. N.Y. Acad. Sci. 252: 124-134.

Prieto, J., Barry, M. and Sherlock, S. 1975. Serum ferritin in patients with iron overload and with acute and chronic liver disease. Gastroenterology 68: 525-533.

Ramsay, J.A., Brown, R.H.J. and Falloon, S.W.H.W. 1953. Simultaneous demonstration of sodium and potassium in small volumes of fluid by flame photometry. J. Exper. Biol. 30: 31.

Raven, J.L., Robson, M.B., Morgan, J.O. and Hoffbrand, A.V. 1971. Comparison of three methods for measuring vitamin B12 in serum: Radioisotopic, Euglena gracilis and Lactobacillus leichmannii. Brit. J. Haematol. 22: 21-31.

Rivers, J.M. and Devine, M.M. 1972. Plasma ascorbic acid concentrations and oral contraceptives. Amer. J. Clin. Nutr. 26: 684-689.

Rodrigo, C., Antezana, C. and Baraona, E. 1971. Fat and nitrogen balances in rats with alcohol-induced fatty liver. J. Nutr. 101: 1307-1310.

Roe, D.A. and Liebman, B. 1977. Folacin intake and status of an elderly institutionalized sample. Fed. Proc. 36: 1121 (Abst.).

Rollason, J.G., Pincherle, C. and Robinson, D. 1972. Serum gamma transpeptidase in relation to alcohol consumption. Clin. Chim. Acta. 39: 75-90.

Rosalki, S.B., Rau, D., Lehmann, D. et al. 1970. Gamma-glutamyl transpeptidase in chronic alcoholism. Lancet 2: 1139.

Rosenthal, W.S., Adham, N.F., Lopez, R. and Cooperman, J.M. 1973. Riboflavin deficiency in complicated chronic alcoholism. Amer. J. Clin. Nutr. 26: 858-860.

Russell, R.I. and Lee, F.D. 1978. Test of small-intestinal function - digestion, absorption, secretion. In Clinics in Gastroenterology. Philadelphia: W.B. Saunders Co. 7: #2. pp. 277-315.

Sarles, H. 1975. Alcohol and the pancreas. Ann. New York Acad. Sci. 252: 171-182.

Sarles, H., Sarles, J.C., Barnatte, R., Muratore, R., Gaini, M., Guren, C., Pastor, J. and Leroy, F. 1965. Observations on 205 confirmed cases of acute pancreatitis and chronic pancreatitis. Gut 6: 545-559.

Sauberlich, H.E. 1975. Vitamin C status: methods and findings. Ann. N.Y. Acad. Sci. 258: 438-450.

Sauberlich, H.E., Dowdy, R.P. and Skala, J.H. 1974. Laboratory Tests for the Assessment of Nutritional Status. Cleveland: CRC Press, Inc. pp. 4-13, 22-30, 70-74.

Shaw, S. and Lieber, C.S. 1977. Alcoholism. In *Nutritional Support of Medical Practice*. Eds. Schneider, H.A., Anderson, C.E. and Coursin, D.B. Hagerstown, MD, New York: Harper and Row. p. 209.

Shaw, S. and Lieber, C.S. 1978. Plasma amino acid abnormalities in the alcoholic. Gastroenterology 74: 677-682.

Sherlock, S. 1955. *Diseases of the Liver and Biliary System*, 3rd ed. Philadelphia: F.A. Davis Co. pp. 16-54.

Sherlock, S. 1963. *Diseases of the Liver*, 3rd ed. Philadelphia: F.A. Davis Co. pp. 115-117, 145-150.

Simmons, W.K. 1972. Urinary urea nitrogen/creatinine ratio as indicator of recent protein intake in field studies. Amer. J. Clin. Nutr. 25: 539-542.

Skeggs, H.R. 1963. Lactobacillus leichmannii assay for vitamin B_{12}. In *Analytical Microbiology*. Ed. Kavanagh, E. New York: Academic Press. p. 551.

Smith, J.C. Jr., McDaniel, E.G., Fan, F.F. and Halsted, J.A. 1973. Zinc: A trace element essential in vitamin A metabolism. Science 181: 954-955.

Spray, G.H. 1968. Oral contraceptives and serum folate levels. Lancet 2: 110.

Teschke, R., Brand, A., and Strohmeyer, G. 1977. Induction of hepatic microsomal gamma-glutamyltransferase activity following chronic alcohol consumption. Biochem. Biophys. Res. Commun. 75: 718-724.

Thompson, A.D., Baker, H. and Leevy, C.M. 1970. Patterns of ^{35}S-thiamine hydrochloride absorption in the malnourished alcoholic patient. J. Lab. Clin. Med. 76: 34-45.

Tillotson, J.A. and Baker, E.M. 1972. An enzymatic measurement of the riboflavin status in man. Amer. J. Clin. Nutr. 25: 425-431.

Tomasulo, P.A. 1968. Impairment of thiamin absorption in alcoholism. Amer. J. Clin. Nutr. 21: 1341-1344.

van de Kamer, J.H., ten Bokkel Huenink, H. and Weyes, H.A. 1949. Rapid method for determination of fat in faeces. J. Biol. Chem. 177: 347-355.

Waldmann, T.A. 1966. Protein-losing enteropathy. Gastroenterology 50: 422-443.

Wands, J.R., Rowe, J.A., Mezey, S.E. *et al.* 1976. Normal serum ferritin concentrations in precirrhotic hemochromatosis. New Eng. J. Med. 294: 302-305.

Wenger, J., Kirsner, J.R. and Palmer, W.L. 1957. Blood carotene in steatorrhoea and the malabsorptive syndromes. Amer. J. Med. 23: 373-380.

Whitfield, J.B., Pounder, R.E., Neale, G. and Moss, D.W. 1972. Serum α-glutamyl transpeptidase activity in liver disease. Gut. 13: 702-708.

Whitehead, T.P., Clarke, C.A. and Whitfield, A.G.W. 1978. Biochemical and haematological markers of alcohol intake. Lancet 1: 978-981.

Whitehead, R.G., Frood, T.D.L. and Poskitt, E.M.E. 1971. Serum albumin measurements in nutritional surveys. A reappraisal. Lancet 2: 287-289.

Willis, J.B. 1965. The analysis of biological materials by atomic absorption spectrometry. Clin. Chem. 11, Suppl., 251-258.

Wilson, F.A. and Dietschy, J.M. 1971. Differential diagnostic approach to clinical problems of malabsorption. Gastroenterology 61: 911-931.

Wormsley, K.G. 1978. Tests of pancreatic secretion. In *Clinics in Gastroenterology*, Vol. 7, #2, Philadelphia: W.B. Saunders Co. p. 529.

10

Nutritional Rehabilitation of Alcoholics

In the nutritional rehabilitation of alcoholics, the goals are five in number:

1. to decrease symptoms and disability of alcohol-related diseases;
2. to prolong and improve the quality of life;
3. to promote capacity for productive work;
4. to reduce the incidence of acute and life-threatening metabolic complications of alcohol abuse; and
5. to modify eating and drinking behavior.

Given that we now have ample evidence that chronic alcohol toxicity produces irreversible tissue damage even when the diet is adequate with respect to macro and micronutrients, faith in nutritional intervention as a means of preventing the development of pathology in such target organs as the liver is misplaced. Further, even under circumstances where modification of the diet or administration of nutrient supplements can reverse alcohol-related malnutrition, a prerequisite for success is that drinking is stopped.

Whereas prerequisites for absolute success in nutritional rehabilitation of alcoholics are abstinence and the reversibility of alcohol-induced tissue damage, certain complications of alcoholism may be prevented or ameliorated by diet. Modifications in lifestyle are essential to nutrition intervention. The more affluent alcoholic who is occupationally or socially exposed to dietary excess, and the indigent alcoholic who subsists on sketchy barroom snacks, are both unlikely candidates for nutritional improvement. The quality of the alcoholic's diet is only as good as the life situation permits, as personal preference dictates, and as medical problems allow.

Nutritional rehabilitation is best initiated under hospital conditions where access to alcoholic beverages is impossible. The treatment plan is the joint responsibility of the nutritionist as well as the patient's physician, the attending nurse, and in many instances, the team should include a pharmacist to give guidance on nutrient supplements. We assume that the first stage of nutritional rehabilitation may be concurrent with the management of alcohol withdrawal. If follow-up is in a residential alcoholism rehabilitation unit, then dietary compliance may be facilitated both by staff and patients' support. The wisdom of discharging the patient from the hospital to return to the previous living situation must be questioned. It is best that the nutritionist and the hospital social worker make an appropriate discharge plan for the patient, which must include arrangement for continued alcoholism counseling on an individual/group/family basis, as well as placement in lodgings with adequate cooking facilities if the family situation is inappropriate, or if breakdown of family relationships has previously taken place.

SECTION 1: NUTRITIONAL MANAGEMENT OF THE ALCOHOLIC IN ACUTE CARE

Food as well as nutrient requirements of alcoholics differ from those of nonalcoholics and within the alcoholics group, requirements vary from times of active drinking to times of abstinence. Diet can modify alcohol-related disorders of the gastrointestinal tract. Alcohol causes acute gastritis with or without nausea, vomiting, and upper abdominal pain. These symptoms persist in the phase after alcohol is withdrawn. The diet should be such as to minimize these symptoms. In acute alcoholic gastritis, hyperchlorhydria is due to a direct stimulant effect of alcohol on gastric acid secretion. There is an ever-present risk in patients with alcoholic gastritis, that peptic ulceration may supervene. Peptic ulcers may be acute or chronic and have either a gastric or duodenal location. Contributory factors related to greater severity of symptoms associated with the gastritis, as well as in the induction of peptic ulceration, include irregular meals, low meal frequency, excess coffee consumption, excessive cigarette smoking, as well as zero or low intake of milk.

In the patient who is under treatment for alcohol abuse either in a detoxication unit or in a clinic or general in-patient hospital situation, cigarette smoking should be prohibited. Unfortunately, this rule is often not followed, and indeed, it is frequent to see alcoholic patients under treatment with cigarette consumption escalating, rather than the reverse. Indeed, no attempt may be made to impose a cigarette ban. Unless cigarette smoking is stopped, it is unlikely that any modification in the eating pattern or the composition of the diet will have a beneficial effect on gastrointestinal effects of alcohol abuse.

In the acute phase of gastritis after a patient has stopped drinking, meals should be small, frequent, and dry, and fluids in the form of water or fruit juices should be given between eating times.

Symptomatic milk intolerance occurs due to temporary lactase deficiency. Milk or milk-containing foods cause gas pain, bloating, and diarrhea. Lactose intolerance is more likely to be present in Blacks than in Whites. Low lactose oral feeding supplements such as Lolactene (Doyle Pharmaceutical Co.) or other similar products are generally well tolerated.

Biochemical assessment of the nutritional status of alcoholics during detoxication is highly recommended as multiple nutritional deficiencies may be present. Dietary prescription must depart from Recommended Dietary Allowances insofar that aims are to combat malnutrition and to guard against metabolic disturbances secondary to alcohol abuse or alcohol related disease (Table 10.1). Therapeutic vitamins and minerals should be prescribed following the protocol summarized in Table 10.2.

In the event that nausea, vomiting or acute alcoholic psychosis hinders or prevents oral feeding, injectable vitamin mixtures should be given. Tube feeding with a low-lactose, high calorie meal replacement formula may be used to provide effective nutritional management and permit anabolism in the patient who cannot retain food by mouth. It is important not to add the required B vitamins to gavage feeding system if evidence is obtained from laboratory tests that the patient has an alcohol-related malabsorption syndrome.

Abnormal pancreatic function occur in a high proportion of chronic alcoholic patients immediately following active drinking. Mezey and Potter (1976) comment that most of these abnormalities will revert to normal after the institution of an adequate diet, whether or not a limited amount of alcohol is also ingested. In a group of five male alcoholic patients, ranging in age from 35 to 61 years, they assessed pancreatic function by means of the pancreozymin-secretin test. Patients were given ethanol at a level of 250 g/day in divided doses. On a low protein (25 g, 1800 kcal) diet, initial impairments in pancreatic function did not improve. When the protein intake was raised to 100 gm/day and the food-energy increased to 2,600 kcal for 10 days, there was a return to normal in the output of bicarbonate, amylase, lipase, and chymotrypsin. Readministration of the low protein diet for 10 days caused a decreased output both of amylase and chymotrypsin. It appears that the temporary dysfunction of the exocrine pancreas which has been seen in actively drinking, chronic alcoholic patients, may be

TABLE 10.1   DIET PRESCRIPTIONS FOR HOSPITALIZED ALCOHOLICS

Patient Profile

Malnutrition with weight loss, muscle wasting and biochemical evidence of multiple vitamin deficiencies and mineral depletion.
Subclinical alcoholic hepatitis.

High energy – moderate protein – high vitamin diet

Food energy

30 kcal/kg/day. Adjust depending on activity. Supplement with IV glucose if nausea, vomiting or anorexia are present.

Nutrients

Protein: Initially 0.5 g/kg/day of high quality protein. Increase to 0.8-1.0 g/kg/day after 5-7 days.

Vitamins: Include vitamin-fortified foods and therapeutic vitamin supplements.

Minerals: Correct electrolyte imbalance. Administer zinc plus magnesium salts.

Foods for the day

	Initial	After 7 days
Milk	120 ml	360 ml
Meat or fish	90 g	180 g
Fruit and fruit juice	6 servings	as for 1st wk.
Low protein vegetables or vegetable juice	2 servings	,,
Fortified breakfast cereal	1 serving	,,
Enriched bread	3 servings	,,
Sugar, jelly, syrup, hard candy, sherbet, margarine		

Number of feedings: 6

caused by deficient dietary protein intake. We therefore advocate that protein intake should be maintained at a level approximately 0.8 g/kg/day provided that biochemical tests do not show gross impairment of liver function with or without hyperammonemia (see treatment of alcoholic liver disease).

Since high fat diets appear also to contribute to the development of alcoholic pancreatitis, there may be some justification for reduction in the fat content of oral feedings. However, it is not conclusively proven that by restricting fat, the recovery of the alcohol-damaged pancreas is hastened.

TABLE 10.2 PROTOCOL FOR VITAMIN-MINERAL THERAPY REQUIRED BY ALCOHOLICS IN ACUTE CARE UNITS

1. If signs and laboratory studies permit diagnosis of defined avitaminoses, treat by administration of individual micronutrients at therapeutic dosage levels.[1]

2. When evidence for specific deficiencies is unclear or incomplete, proceed to the following routine:

   a) On admission, give single i.m. dose of 100 mg thiamin (Thiamine hydrochloride USP solution, 100 mg/ml).

   b) If macrocytic (megaloblastic) anemia is present, check vitamin B_{12} status before prescribing folic acid greater than RDA.

   c) Give daily water soluble and fat soluble vitamins in hospital mixture based on approximately the following dosages: thiamin mononitrate 15 mg; riboflavin 15 mg; pyridoxine hydrochloride 25 mg; niacinamide 100 mg; cyanocobalamin 5 μg; folic acid 1.5 mg; ascorbic acid 200 mg; vitamin A 5000 i.u.; vitamin D 400 i.u. and vitamin E 30 i.u.[2].

   d) Correct electrolyte imbalance and magnesium deficiency by i.v. mineral solutions.

   e) If zinc deficiency is clearly present or suspected give zinc sulfate 300 mg daily.

---

[1]Phytonadione (vitamin K_1) may be required to treat vitamin K deficiency with hypoprothrobinemia prior to surgery. Usual preparation should be AquaMephyton 15 mg/m.

[2]Proprietary therapeutic vitamin preparations do not conform with the composition of recommended mixture. Acceptable commercial formulations of water soluble vitamins are Berocca tabs (Roche) or Larobec (Roche), which should be given (1 tab daily) with a fat soluble vitamin preparation such as Decavitamin U.S.P.

SECTION 2 : NUTRITIONAL SUPPORT OF THE ALCOHOLIC IN SURGERY

The chronic alcoholic is a high risk patient when s/he has to undergo surgical procedures. Special hazards and their underlying nutritional or metabolic causes are listed in Table 10.3.

Nutritional management of the alcoholic patient before and after surgery requires knowledge of the risks, an ability to recognize presenting syndromes and experience in modern methods of nutritional support (Table 10.4).

Several presenting nutritional syndromes require special discussion because they are not well described in standard medical textbooks, and because unless they are recognized early and treated, they are life threatening. These syndromes arise because standard preoperative and/or postoperative food withdrawal allows alcoholics, in previously marginal nutritional status, to develop overt signs of deficiencies.

TABLE 10.3 PRE- AND POST-OPERATIVE NUTRITIONAL/METABOLIC HAZARDS OF SURGERY IN THE ALCOHOLIC

Classification	Presenting Syndrome	Causal Mechanism
Electrolyte imbalance	Potassium depletion	Vomiting, diarrhea Hyperaldosteronism Muscle wasting Renal tubular acidosis Diuretics
	Sodium/water retention	Portal hypertension Hypoalbuminemia Altered renal hemodynamics Endocrine dysfunction (adrenal) Changes in lymph flow
Metabolic crises	Hypoglycemia	Impaired gluconeogenesis Glycogen depletion Starvation
	Keto acidosis Hepatic encephalopathy (Hyperammonemia)	Starvation/ethanol Hepatic failure Porto-caval shunts
	Gout (Hyperuricemia)	Starvation Ethanol

Alcohol withdrawal	Seizures
	Hallucinosis
	Delirium tremens
		Quantity of alcohol pre-
		  viously ingested
		Rate of termination of
		  drinking episode
		Rebound excitation
		Hypomagnesemia
		Respiratory alkalosis

Malnutrition a) pre-operative	Chronic protein- energy malnutrition (adult marasmus)	Inadequate protein-energy intake, anorexia, etc. Maldigestion Low vitamin intake
	Avitaminoses (Wernicke-Korsakoff) and other thiamin syndrome deficiencies	Malabsorption Impaired vitamin utilization
b) post-operative	Visceral protein attrition	Food withdrawal; Catabolic stress
	Protein malnutrition (combined type) Zinc deficiency	Severe catabolic stress + pre-operative marasmus Prolonged IV feeding Hyperexcretion Zn
	Delayed wound healing	Protein, vitamin C & zinc deficiency
	Sepsis	Impaired cellular immunity associated w/protein malnu- trition

TABLE 10.3 (*Continued*)

Classification	Presenting Syndrome	Causal Mechanism
	Anemia	Blood loss Folacin deficiency B6 deficiency
	Confusional psychosis	Niacin deficiency
Adverse reactions to anesthesia	Hepatic failure	Combined alcoholic liver damage, halothane and protein malnutrition

TABLE 10.4 NUTRITIONAL MANAGEMENT OF ALCOHOLIC SURGICAL PATIENTS

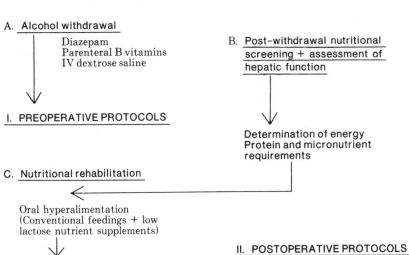

A. Alcohol withdrawal

    Diazepam
    Parenteral B vitamins
    IV dextrose saline

B. Post-withdrawal nutritional
    screening + assessment of
    hepatic function

I. PREOPERATIVE PROTOCOLS

Determination of energy
Protein and micronutrient
requirements

C. Nutritional rehabilitation

Oral hyperalimentation
(Conventional feedings + low
lactose nutrient supplements)

II. POSTOPERATIVE PROTOCOLS

D. Immediate preoperative nutrition
    intervention

Oral Gatorade or Citrotein (Doyle)
IV dextrose saline
Parenteral B vitamins
Vitamin C and Vitamin K

E. Postoperative nutritional
    screening and monitoring

F. Fluid and electrolytes IV

G. Chemically defined diet—oral,
    (low lactose)   intragastric

H. Oral hyperalimentation

I. Total parenteral alimentation
   with complicated trauma or
   surgery

In the case of emergency surgery,
omit C and after BRIEF nutritional
screening employ combined A+D proto-
cals.
Successive post-operative feeding
protocols all require addition of
parenteral B vitamins and vitamin C
and zinc initially IV and orally
as soon as oral feeds are restarted.

While visceral protein malnutrition occurs as a post-operative disorder, protein-energy malnutrition is most frequent in non-alcoholics who have been denied food in the pre-operative period and have then been subjected to the catabolic stress of surgical procedures, it is more common, more severe and more likely to be complicated by peripheral protein malnutrition in alcoholics. Diagnosis is on the basis of depressed serum proteins, including serum albumin and transferrin as well as evidence of depressed cellular immune function. In the alcoholic this kwashiorkor-like form of protein malnutrition is characterized by edema, particularly of the wound area which fails to heal. Postoperatively, alcoholics tend also to exhibit this condition in combination with progressive wasting. Wound sepsis and septicemia induced by gram-negative microorganism may supervene unless nutritional intervention is prompt. Blackburn and Bistrian (1977) recommend restoration of protein status if visceral protein malnutrition (attrition) by a protein sparing routine and stress that peripheral protein malnutrition (adult marasmus) patients should receive daily energy and protein feedings at levels to meet their requirements. However, in the alcoholic with hepatitis or cirrhosis, the advantages of rapid protein repletion must be weighed against the risks of hepatic encephalopathy induced by exceeding nitrogen tolerance.

Zinc deficiency may develop in an alcoholic during the post-operative period because of longstanding hyperzincuria, recent catabolic stress with muscle wasting, and infusion of IV fluids which do not contain zinc salts. Classical signs include acrodermatitis, or a scaly red rash which spreads from the extremities to the trunk. Failure for the operative wound to epithelialize is a cardinal feature. Loss of taste is common once the patient has been allowed to commence oral feeding. Variants of the syndrome may occur with symptoms of psychosis in some patients including antisocial attitudes and disorientation. Diagnosis is from serum zinc measurements. In zinc deficiency, serum zinc levels are uniformly low. Response to zinc salts by the oral or IV routes is prompt with complete resolution. The dermatosis clears, taste sensation returns and mental symptoms disappear. Oral zinc sulfate therapy should be at a level of 300 mg/day (Tucker et al., 1976; Ecker and Schroiter, 1978).

Syndromes of acute niacin deficiency were described by the late Grace Goldsmith (1977). The first of these syndromes is characterized by confusion, disorientation and hallucinations resembling an acute toxic psychosis. The other was described as an acute encephalopathy with stupor, cogwheel rigidity of the extremities, as well as grasping and sucking reflexes. In the author's experience, these patients are easily roused in response to the spoken voice, but soon relapse with partial loss of consciousness. Both syndromes were said to occur in "malnourished subjects following IV administration of glucose without concomitant administration of niacin." Niacinamide, 50 mg every 8 hours (q8h) orally is recommended as treatment or niacinamide can be given by the IV route since unlike niacin, it does not produce vasodilatation.

Although Goldsmith did not describe these syndromes as post-operative complications in alcoholics, alcoholics do develop these syndromes and risk is highest in the post-surgical period. Response to niacinamide may not, in the author's experience, be as prompt as Goldsmith claimed, particularly with the second syndrome. Delayed response to nutritional intervention may be because of late effects of phenothiazine or benzodiazepine tranquilizers or to the concurrent presence of thiamin deficiency.

Decreased synthesis of clotting factors II (prothrombin), VII, IX, and X in alcoholics with hepatitis or cirrhosis enhances the post-operative risk of wound hemorrhage. Since synthesis of these clotting factors is vitamin K-dependent, and vitamin K deficiency may exist in alcoholics due both to deficient intake and malabsorption, a vitamin K preparation should be given preoperatively if the prothrombin time is prolonged or other clotting tests are abnormal. However, in advanced alcoholic liver disease, there may be a hepatic parenchymal defect in the synthesis of these clotting factors which is not correctable by vitamin K (Mezey, 1978).

SECTION 3: RECENT ADVANCES IN NUTRITIONAL THERAPY OF CHRONIC ALCOHOLICS

A. Nightblindness: The Need for Vitamin A and Zinc

Marginal vitamin A status or frank vitamin A deficiency with night-blindness occurs commonly in alcoholics with cirrhosis. It has been shown by Russell et al. (1978) that vitamin A therapy, or vitamin A plus zinc, improves dark adaptation and vitamin A status in male cirrhotics. A group of 26 men with mild to moderate alcoholic cirrhosis was studied with respect to dark adaptation thresholds and biochemical assessment of vitamin A status was estimated from measurements of plasma retinol, retinyl esters, retinol-binding, and prealbumin. The serum zinc and fecal fat were also measured. The investigator found that 15 men in the group had dark adaptation abnormalities (elevated thresholds). Patients with impairment of dark adaptation tended to have lower levels of plasma retinol binding protein, and prealbumin, but levels were not significantly reduced in comparison with the remaining patients who had normal dark adaptation. Serum zinc concentrations were low in three patients with abnormal dark adaptation, but within the normal range in the other patients. Fat malabsorption was present in seven patients with, and in seven patients without, abnormalities of dark adaptation.

The aim of the three treatment plans was to normalize dark adaptation. Twelve of the 14 patients with abnormal dark adaptation received oral, water-miscible retinyl palmitate at a dose of 3,300 μg/day for 2-4 weeks. In the patients whose dark adaptation threshold remained elevated after this treatment, oral retinyl palmitate at a level of 3,300 μg/day plus zinc sulfate 220 mg/day was given if baseline zinc levels were in the normal range. Treatments were discontinued if dark adaptation returned to normal.

Among the 12 treated patients, 8 responded to the initial lower dose vitamin A therapy, two who were initially zinc deficient responded to further vitamin A plus zinc sulfate, and the remaining two who received the higher dose of vitamin A showed abnormal dark adaptation at the end of the study (one of these patients had fat malabsorption). Biochemical changes with vitamin A therapy included an increase in plasma retinol, retinyl esters, and retinol-binding protein. It is suggested that administration of vitamin A to alcoholics with cirrhosis can stimulate the release of retinol binding protein. We are also reminded that zinc stimulates synthesis of retinol binding protein. However, in two patients who received zinc in addition to vitamin A, plasma retinol and retinol binding protein did not further increase, suggesting to the author that zinc had a direct effect on the retina, perhaps stimulating alcohol dehydrogenase activity in the conversion of retinal from retinol. Experience has shown that when infants or young children with protein-calorie malnutrition are refed with diets which do not contain vitamin A, vitamin A deficiency may be precipitated. Therapeutic lessons for the treatment of malnourished or cirrhotic alcoholics, to be gained from the Russell study, are that nutritional rehabilitation programs for chronic alcoholics should include vitamin A and zinc supplementations.

B. B Vitamins in Alcoholic Neuropathy and Brain Syndromes

In a study of chronic alcoholics by Datsun *et al.* (1976), patients with peripheral neuropathy, confusion and disorientation were found not only to have decreased blood levels of thiamin and low erythrocyte transketolase activity, but also biochemical evidence of riboflavin, niacin, folacin and pyridoxine deficiency. Low levels of thiamin, riboflavin, niacin and pyridoxine were found in the cerebrospinal fluid. Low CSF levels of thiamin, niacin and pyridoxine were found more frequently in patients with mental changes than in those who only had peripheral neuropathy.

We are reminded that a functional interrelationship exists between the B vitamins and that thiamin, niacin, pyridoxine and folacin deficiencies can produce neurological signs. From the therapeutic standpoint, it is advisable to treat malnourished alcoholics, particularly those with neurological defects as well as liver disease, with a pharmacological combination of these B vitamins. However, whether this will allow resolution of neuropathy or encephalopathy will also depend on alcohol withdrawal and on whether neural damage is due to toxic effects of ethanol per se or to deficiency of one or more B vitamins or to a state of vitamin dependency.

C. Management of Iron Overload

Iron overload can be suspected in alcoholics who have excess iron in plasma cells seen in bone marrow smears. Chronic alcoholic patients with a history of anemia, cirrhosis, hepatitis, pancreatitis, and pulmonary tuberculosis, described by Karcioglu and Hardison (1978), had excessive bone marrow iron stores and iron-containing plasma cells. Iron overload in these patients was due either to excessive intake, hyperabsorption or malutilization because of folacin and pyridoxine deficiencies.

Editorial comment on management of iron overload in such chronic alcoholics is to the effect that patients should be warned not to eat iron-fortified foods (Editorial, Nutr. Rev., 1978). We would also advocate vitamin B and folacin to correct anemia due to deficiency of these vitamins and that caution should be exercised in selecting appropriate drug therapy for coexistent pulmonary tuberculosis. Several drugs used in the treatment of this disease, including notably isonicotinic acid hydrazide (Isoniazid, INH), and cycloserine, are vitamin B_6 antagonists and can cause sideroblastic anemia (Roe, 1976).

SECTION 4: PROPHYLAXIS AND TREATMENT OF ACUTE METABOLIC CRISES IN ALCOHOLICS

Acute metabolic disturbances in actively drinking alcoholics which require emergency treatment include hypoglycemia, metabolic acidosis and in patients with genetically-determined intermittent porphyria, acute attacks of this disease. Attacks of gout may also be precipitated by alcohol abuse.

Hypoglycemia, metabolic acidosis and acute porphyria attacks are all precipitated by fasting. Despite problems with compliance, it is therefore the duty of physicians, nutritionists, and other health care personnel, charged with the responsibility of alcoholic patients, to warn them, in lay language, of the life-threatening situations which may arise if they drink continuously without consuming any food. Further, emergency room MD's and nurses as well as surgeons and anesthetists need to be constantly aware of the high risk of hypoglycemia and/or metabolic acidosis developing in alcoholics who are denied energy intake after injury as well as pre- and post-surgery.

When an alcoholic cannot tolerate oral feeding, or when oral feeding is denied for reasons of surgical management or if hypoglycemia, metabolic acidosis or attacks of acute porphyria are present, the life-saving measures are dextrose infusion and correction of electrolyte imbalance. In a report on treatment outcome with different modalities in alcoholic acidosis (Miller *et al.,* 1978), it was found that improvement was faster with intravenous administration of dextrose (7.0-7.5 g/hr) than with IV saline. There was a more rapid decline in absolute levels of B-hydroxybutyrate and acetoacetate as well as the ratio between these metabolites. Plasma-free fatty acid levels declined. Patients who received phosphate also improved rapidly, but the authors were not convinced that phosphate infusion significantly altered outcome. They postulated that with glucose or phosphate administration, phosphorus levels within hepatocytes increased, and mitochondrial oxidation of NADH to NAD is induced.

Since ethanol-induced hyperuricemia with acute gouty arthritis can also be precipitated by fasting (Maclachlan and Rodman, 1967), the alcoholic with a history of gout, should be advised that attack frequency can be reduced by increasing the frequency of food intake. Again, physicians having alcoholics as patients in acute care hospitals should be reminded that acute gout may develop if starvation is imposed.

SECTION 5 : NUTRITIONAL SUPPORT DURING ALCOHOL WITHDRAWAL

Principles of management during alcohol withdrawal include psychological intervention, sedation, nutritional support and special treatment of complications. Outcome is improved by following preset protocols for patients' assessment and therapeutic plans.

In the initial assessment, rapid but precise screening of patients is essential to determine:

a. nutritional status;
b. presence or absence of metabolic complications of alcohol abuse (hypoglycemia/ketoacidosis); and
c. characteristics of specific alcohol withdrawal syndrome if present.

These procedures must be carried out in addition to routine medical screening and examination for signs of injury or infection.

Nutritional assessment should be a) clinical (evidence of dehydration, wasting, edema, as well as cutaneous and neurological signs of avitaminoses); b) dietary: the patient is usually unreliable concerning his/her dietary history. Information sources, other than the patient, may be family members, other household members, and drinking companions. Needs of the physician/nutritionist are to find out if the patient has been entirely without food and if so, for how long, and secondly the general eating pattern prior to the most recent debauch.

Anthropometric assessment should include height, weight, triceps skinfold thickness, and mid upper arm circumference.

Biochemical assessment should include blood alcohol level, routine serum electrolytes, serum magnesium and zinc, erythrocyte transketolase (for thiamin status), blood glucose, including sodium, potassium, chloride and bicarbonate, serum transaminases (SGOT, SGPT), serum bilirubin, blood urea nitrogen, serum creatinine, serum albumin, serum transferrin and plasma plus erythrocyte folacin.

Nutritional support is an essential component of total management. Management should follow guidelines set by Leigh Thompson (1978). Patients who do not display clinical or biochemical signs of malnutrition should be under observation lest nausea, vomiting or anorexia during the withdrawal period leads to refusal of food and liquids and hence rapid development of dehydration, acute protein-energy malnutrition, and B vitamin-dependent syndromes. We recognize that for all patients during withdrawal, sedation with a benzodiazepine tranquilizer (diazepam 5-10 mg q4-q6h) should be combined with therapeutic vitamin preparation which can be given orally or parenterally, depending on whether substances given by mouth can be retained. The thiamin supplement should be set at a minimal level of 100 mg/day and folic acid at 1.5 mg/day.

If the patient is dehydrated and/or unable to tolerate oral feeds, dextrose saline should be given intravenously with addition of thiamin 100 mg q12h and other therapeutic vitamins according to results of nutritional assessment. Vitamin levels for IV administration, with the exception of thiamin, can follow the formulation suggested by Shils (1972) and adopted by Meng (1977) in total parenteral hyperalimentation when biochemical assessment of vitamin status is not readily available. Electrolyte imbalance must be corrected; particular attention being paid to reversal of hypokalemia and hypomagnesemia.

When hallucinoses or major motor seizures (rumfits) occur, priority is for the arrest of seizures by giving diazepam IV, mg 5 q5-15 min followed by diazepam orally or IV mg 5-15 q2-q6h.

If the patient exhibits the signs of delirium tremens with extreme autonomic hyperactivity, sweating, tachycardia, insomnia, confusion, delusions and characteristic hallucinations, management should be as for other conditions requiring intensive care, with continuous monitoring of vital signs. Diazepam should be given 5 mg q5min IV until patient is sedated, and then 5-15 mg q2-q6h. With either the complication of hallucinosis, seizures, or delirium tremens, therapy should include hydration, dextrose administration, correction of electrolyte imbalance and administration of pharmacologic doses of thiamin are required as in the management of other dehydrated or food intolerant alcoholics during withdrawal.

SECTION 6 : ALCOHOLIC LIVER DISEASE

Alcohol abuse leads to liver damage which may be reversible or irreversible. It has been made clear that no phase in the development of alcoholic liver disease, from fatty liver to hepatitis and from hepatitis to cirrhosis can be prevented by intake of a single nutrient or a combination of nutrients. Indeed, as intimated by Lieber (1975), the hope of the alcoholic that a particular dietary regime or vitamin preparation can be protective against progressive liver injury, while heavy drinking is continued, should be dispelled both by the physician and by the nutritionist.

A. Alcoholic Steatosis

From the prophylactic standpoint, it is recognized that a low fat diet does diminish the degree of fatty liver or steatosis that develops in human volunteers for given levels of alcohol intake (Lieber and Spritz, 1966). Similarly, in rats given liquid diets of adequate protein content, with varying amounts of fat, reduction in the fat content of the animals' diet to 25% or less of total energy intake is associated with a diminution in the degree of steatosis induced by alcohol (Lieber and De-Carli, 1970). Further, Lieber et al. (1967) have shown that not only the level of fat intake but also the chain length of dietary fatty acids are important for the degree of steatosis after experimental alcohol feeding. At least in the rat, when dietary triglycerides containing long chain fatty acids are replaced by a fat source containing medium chain triglycerides the occurrence of fatty liver is reduced.

In order to explain these findings, Lieber and DeCarli (1977) have suggested that the advantage of feeding medium chain fatty acids is based on their metabolic biotransformation by oxidation rather than esterification.

Partial protection against alcoholic steatosis has also been produced by administration of agents which reduce hyperlipemia including the drug chlorophenoxyisobutyrate (Atromid S) (Spritz and Lieber, 1966; Brown, 1966), and niacin (Baker et al., 1973).

Niacin treatment prevented the accumulation of non-esterified fatty acids, total lipids, and neutral lipids in the livers of rats given ethanol.

The question which remains unanswered is whether fat reduction, or modification in the fat source of the drinkers' diet, or administration of niacin supplements, alters prognosis with respect to the progression of alcoholic steatosis to irreversible liver damage. Our practical application of knowledge of the effects of dietary lipid and lipid status on the drinkers' liver is to caution the binge drinker to reduce intake of fats and to provide a fat-restricted diet to alcoholics under treatment in acute or long-term care units. Since there is no evidence that niacin supplementation does prevent or delay alcoholic liver disease except in laboratory animals and because megadoses of niacin are toxic, we do not recommend that pharmacologic doses of niacin are appropriate in the routine management of alcoholics.

B. Alcoholic Hepatitis, Cirrhosis, and Hepatic Encephalopathy

Nutritional support is appropriate and justifiable to reverse malnutrition which is a consequence of alcoholic liver disease and to minimize the risk of acute, potentially fatal metabolic disturbances which complicate alcoholic hepatitis and cirrhosis. Clinical experience further suggests that if an alcoholic stops drinking on a permanent basis, then return of specific liver functions towards normality is promoted by nutritional rehabilitation. Indeed, there is evidence to support the assumption that reparative activity within the hepatocytes is enhanced by nutritional support. Mezey (1978) has pointed out that with liver injury, whether from ethanol or other toxins, nitrogen requirements are increased to provide for liver regeneration and that unless the nitrogen is available from the diet, it will be drawn from other organs leading, it is assumed, to peripheral protein malnutrition. Increases in plasma glucagon as well as decreases in plasma insulin to glucagon ratio contribute to stepped up gluconeogenesis with release of amino acids from muscle. According to Mezey, this may lead to muscle wasting. Also, plasma amino acid patterns are abnormal in alcoholic liver disease with increases in the concentrations of those amino acids which are normally metabolized by the liver. Amino acids, exceeding the renal threshold, may spill over into the urine, though these nitrogen losses are seldom if ever sufficient to justify increases in dietary nitrogen.

A critical decision on the nutritional management of the alcoholic with liver disease is the appropriate level of nitrogen in the diet and the best protein or amino acid sources. On the one hand, it is necessary to avoid protein malnutrition and exacerbation of endogenous amino acid aberrations and on the other hand, the need is to avoid the development of hepatic encephalopathy. Whereas in patients with advanced liver disease, nitrogen balance may be maintained on a dietary protein intake of 0.5 g/kg/day, the question is whether a positive nitrogen balance reflects attainment of nitrogen requirements since distribution is abnormal. Decreased urea synthesis and accumulations of ammonia leading to hyperammonemia and hepatic encephalopathy reduces the dietary protein tolerance of the alcoholic with alcoholic hepatitis with or without cirrhosis.

It has been found that diets containing protein from non-meat sources are better tolerated by cirrhotics who already have early signs of hepatic encephalopathy with hyperammonemia (Fenton et al., 1966). Among dietary amino acids, methionine is known to precipitate hepatic encephalopathy if fed in high dosage (Phear et al., 1956). Since vegetable protein sources contain less methionine than meat proteins (Rudman et al., 1970), it was considered by Greenberger et al. (1977) that they would be better tolerated by alcoholics with chronic hepatic encephalopathy. Three patients with cirrhosis, porto-caval shunts and chronic recurrent hepatic encephalopathy were studied while on vegetable and animal protein diets, both at levels of approximately 40 g/day. The vegetable protein diet, containing cereals and legumes, and with a total protein content of 41.8 g/day, resulted in clinical improvement, decreased signs of hepatic encephalopathy, lowered blood ammonia level, and better performance with intellectual tasks. In one patient an increase in protein intake was gradually carried out to a final level of 90 g/day without return of symptoms. However, it is difficult to evaluate results of the vegetable protein diet in this patient since lactulose* was also administered. Further confirmation of these find-

---

*Lactulose is a synthetic disaccharide containing galactose and fructose which is neither absorbed nor metabolized. This disaccharide has a beneficial effect on the course of hepatic encephalopathy probably because it has an ammonia-trapping effect in the intestine (Elkington et al., 1969; Bircher et. al., 1971).

ings is needed before the vegetable protein diet is applied to the management of patients with advanced alcoholic liver disease since certainly two out of the three cases described had irreversible liver disease of nonalcoholic etiology.

Protective effects of the vegetable protein diet could be due to the lower methionine content but are more likely due either to changes induced in the intestinal microflora leading to a lessening of ammonia production or to decreased bioavailability of the nitrogen from the vegetable protein.

Neomycin administration, which is the standard drug therapy for hepatic encephalopathy, exerts its therapeutic effect by gut "sterilization." Enteric microflora, responsible for ammonia production from nitrogenous substrates, are inhibited. However, neomycin, at the dosage level required to exert this desired effect, causes maldigestion and malabsorption. Steatorrhea and disaccharide intolerance develop and with chronic administration of neomycin, drug-induced increases in fecal nitrogen losses and impaired absorption of fat-soluble vitamins, including particularly vitamins A, D, and K, can precipitate or exacerbate protein-energy malnutrition and multiple avitaminoses (Thompson et al., 1971; Faloon, 1970).

When, in order to avert or control hepatic encephalopathy, neomycin is given to the alcoholic with hepatitis or cirrhosis, preliminary nutritional assessment is essential and periodic nutritional monitoring should be carried out during the drug regime. The profile of nutritional screening tests should include daily anthropometric measurements consisting in total body weight, triceps skinfold thickness, and mid upper arm circumference, from which body fat and lean muscle mass can be assessed. Records should be kept of change in body weight with treatment as well as change in skinfold thickness and arm muscle mass indicating loss or gain of subcutaneous fat and lean body mass, respectively. In addition, it is recommended that fecal fat determinations and prothrombin times be carried out biweekly as screening tests for malabsorption and associated vitamin K deficiency. When laboratory facilities permit, plasma carotene and retinol as well as plasma 25-hydroxycholecalciferol should be measured. These assessments of nutritional status will enable the physician in charge and the nutritionist, to modify the diet and to give pharmacologic doses of fat soluble vitamins at an appropriate dosage level. It is recommended that fat-soluble vitamins be administered parenterally since adequate intestinal absorption cannot be insured.

Whether the alcoholic with incipient or actual hepatic encephalopathy is treated by a low protein diet alone or a low protein diet with lactulose or neomycin, nitrogen requirements may not be met without recourse to parenteral alimentation. A regime of parenteral alimentation with special amino acids high in branched chain acids but low in aromatic amino acids has been developed. Success with this method of nutritional support has been achieved insofar that neurological status has been improved and there has been an increased survival rate of dogs with porto-caval shunts and some patients with hepatic encephalopathy. Concurrently, normalization of plasma amino acids has been achieved (Rudman et al., 1973).

The theoretical basis for infusion of branched chain amino acids, as a nitrogen source, is that aromatic amino acids and more particularly tryptophan, are involved in the pathogenesis of hepatic coma. Elevated plasma-free tryptophan levels have been found in hepatic coma patients. In a study by Ono et al. (1978), the theory is developed that increased turnover of brain serotonin in patients with hepatic encephalopathy could be related to increased plasma tryptophan levels since this amino acid is the serotonin precursor, and the relative concentration of tryptophan in the plasma may regulate serotonin synthesis or at least the amount of tryptophan entering the brain. The investigators also found that tryptophan levels were significantly increased in patients with cirrhosis and in those with hepatic coma. Plasma phenylalanine, tyrosine and methionine were also increased in coma patients and in the CSF of cirrhosis and coma patients. It is suggested that the biochemical phenomenon observed reflect "a generalized increase in the transport of amino acids across the blood-brain barrier in chronic liver disease." However, since they only found differences in tryptophan concentration between the CSF samples from cirrhotic patients and those from patients in hepatic coma, and no differences in levels of other aromatic amino acids, their hypothesis, quoted above, is not supported.

On the basis of the theory that hepatic coma is related to a disorder of serotonin metabolism with abnormal neurotransmitter function, and with the support of their experimental findings, the investigators suggest a therapeutic approach might be by using agents which reduce the level of tryptophan within the central nervous system.

Several alternate explanations have been offered for the observed benefits obtained from infusion of branched chain amino acid mixtures in patients with hepatic encephalopathy. Presently a conservative viewpoint is that these mixtures offset hyperammonemia as do other therapeutic modalities which have been successful in combatting cerebral effects of liver failure.

Nutritional support of patients with hepatic encephalopathy has also been attempted by administration of keto analogues of the essential amino acids. Maddrey and his coworkers (1976) gave the keto analogues of valine, leucine, isoleucine, methionine, and phenylalanine either parenterally or orally in various proportions to 11 patients with hepatic encephalopathy. Plasma concentrations of the essential amino acids corresponding to these keto analogues increased after infusions. Blood ammonia (arterial) was not significantly altered immediately after IV administration of the keto analogues, but a decrease in whole blood glutamine was observed. Consistent improvement in nitrogen balance was not obtained. Eight of the eleven patients showed clinical improvement as determined by objective neurological and psychological screening. There were no toxic side effects from the regimen.

Essential amino acids can be synthesized from their keto analogues in human subjects as well as in experimental rats. Indeed, nitrogen balance has been maintained when keto analogues of essential amino acids, lacking in the diet, are administered. In these circumstances, ammonia formed in the intestine is a nitrogen source for amino acid synthesis and hepatic glutamine is also a major nitrogen donor (Richards et al., 1967; Walser et al., 1973).

In a recent review by Richards (1978), it has been pointed out that the extent to which keto analogues can replace essential amino acids depends on several dietary factors as well as in the route of administration of the keto analogue. For example, the amount of tyrosine in the diet is the major factor which determines the efficiency by which phenylpyruvate can replace phenylalanine. Further nitrogen balance is highly influenced by energy intake being improved as energy intake is increased. The efficiency of the keto analogues also depends on their rate and degree of absorption.

Advantages of infusing branched chain keto analogues have been shown by Sapir and Walser (1977), who found that these analogues had a positive effect on protein anabolism.

The nutritional management of patients with alcoholic liver disease is summarized in Table 10.5.

SECTION 7 : FOOD BEHAVIOR MODIFICATION – A PROPOSED TREATMENT MODALITY

Within the total framework of alcoholism rehabilitation, promotion of positive change in eating behavior should receive priority. Commonly the alcoholic is a multiple substance abuser. Lack of interest in food and lack of appetite for food are frequently associated with excessive coffee consumption and heavy smoking as well as use of

TABLE 10.5 NUTRITIONAL MANAGEMENT OF ALCOHOLIC LIVER DISEASE

Steatosis ———⟶ Mild Hepatitis　　　　Severe Hepatitis　　　　Cirrhosis

Low fat, moderate protein diet　　　　Low fat, low protein, high carbohydrate diet　　　　Moderate protein, high carbohydrate diet

Acute hepatic encephalopathy

Parenteral alimentation
with
　a) infusion of branched
　　chain amino acids
or　b) keto analogues of
　　essential amino acid

Chronic hepatic encephalopathy

Low protein (veg. protein)
high carbohydrate diet
+ lactulose or neomycin

All diets or intravenous nutrition prescriptions must include therapeutic vitamins (see Table 10.2).

In cirrhosis with ascites, sodium restriction may be required.

prescription, over-the-counter, and illicit drugs. Indeed, we have obtained objective evidence of sick role behavior, particularly among binge drinkers through psychometric tests which suggest not only activities productive of ill health are used as a coping mechanism, but also that symptoms produced by these practices give the individual a desired excuse from work in the home and in the place of employment (Roe, 1978). The antithesis of the sick role is the pursuit of health, which includes betterment of nutritional status through control of self-abusive behavior.

In treatment facilities for alcoholics, where counseling techniques are employed to overcome personal and situational factors which contribute to alcohol abuse, it is common to find that patients rely on cigarette smoking, coffee drinking, candy chewing, as well as their prescribed medications, to overcome anxiety and depression.

Aims of long-range nutrition programs for alcoholics are:
a. Replacement of self-abusive behaviors by health-seeking behavior;
b. Education of patients to understand how food choice can become a health seeking behavior;
c. Upgrading actual eating practices; and
d. Demonstration that appropriate food consumption is a major factor in the acquisition of physical fitness and capacity for work.

In an alcoholism rehabilitation hospital or unit, needs are for a health educator/nutritionist who has had formal training and experience in behavior modification methods. Depending on the staffing patterns and program of the unit the health educator/nutritionist may be assisted by the following health professionals: physicians, nurse-clinicians, nurses, physical therapists, occupational therapists, psychiatric social workers, vocational counselors, as well as members of the dietary department.

Program development requires a motivational approach with emphasis on the undesirable behavior (drinking, smoking, drugs) and the desired behaviors (food-related activity, cessation of smoking, exercise). Desired behavior is rewarded. Staff act as role models. Experiences of the desired behavior are offered, including audiovisual aids. Nutrition education materials should be used as reinforcement at the therapy sessions. These should be geared to the education level of the patients, and should focus on goals of long-term nutritional rehabilitation in the alcoholic. The program should be available to all patients in residence who no longer exhibit signs of alcohol withdrawal. Initial nutritional screening is essential, and patients should be acquainted with finding and recommendations for nutritional rehabilitation. Screening for physical capacity is also necessary. Metabolic responses to exercise are abnormal in chronic alcoholics. Chalmers *et al.* (1977) showed that with exercise, abstinent alcoholics increased blood levels of lactate and pyruvate, had higher blood glycerol levels, and exhibited post-exercise ketosis. Findings suggest insufficient or abnormal utilization of body fuels. We note, however, that the metabolic changes found in the alcoholics included in the study were similar to those of untrained, unfit people.

Diminished exercise tolerance in the alcoholic may be due to alcoholic myopathy, cardiomyopathy, anemia, or any combination of these alcohol-related diseases. It may also be associated with obesity and commonly, it is due to excessive smoking and physical inactivity. The cause(s) should be identified. A program goal is to encourage patients to associate improved eating behavior with greater physical fitness and increased ability to participate in physical exercise.

We recognize that in placing program emphasis on change in physical fitness as an outcome of change in drinking/eating/smoking behavior, caution should be exercised in accepting a single element of this intervention as the cause of health improvement.

In replacing self-abusive behaviors with health seeking behavior we assume a multivariant program with concurrent diet counseling, graduated anti-smoking-exercise facets. Each facet of the program needs to be developed through behavior modification techniques. Patients must be made aware of why they drink excessively, why they eat irregularly, when they smoke and why they have poor exercise tolerance. Substitution of health serving behavior is essential.

With young alcoholics, we have found a ready acceptance of meal planning and preparation as a substitute activity. Interest in the nutritional advantages of food diversity and in meals providing foods of high nutrient to calorie ratios can be conveyed. Further, if these patients are permitted to play an active role in providing food for themselves and for other patients they can become sufficiently occupied with this activity to overcome boredom and to see their food-related occupation as a viable alternate to their previous health abusive practices. In alcoholism units in rural locations, an added dimension is the promotion of home gardens, where vegetables can be grown by patients, and used in the kitchen of the facility.

Whereas it may be advantageous to use behavior modification techniques to motivate alcoholics to seek after health, through change in their food-related practices, this should not be interpreted to mean that excessive eating is better than alcohol abuse. We have seen alcoholic patients who overeat during rehabilitation and as an accompaniment to a sedentary life, this leads to obesity. As Hillman (1974) observed the problem, "Obesity should be particularly guarded against; special precautions are required during the period of early rehabilitation, when patients are particularly at risk of 'rebound overeating'."

Older chronic alcoholics are less likely to be motivated to change their food habits and indeed, program participation by this group is usually irregular. We agree with Anderson (1971), who commented: "They resist efforts to change their life patterns and frequently revert to former over-indulgence in alcohol following the imposed disciplines of hospitalization..."

There is justification in providing a nutrition education program for alcoholics who will benefit from alcoholism rehabilitation to the extent that prognosis is for long or moderately long periods of sobriety. Given that these individuals learn their special nutritional needs, they may be motivated to consume a prudent diet and to take regular vitamin supplements during the periods when they are not drinking. Thereby, their health will benefit and the risk of malnutrition will be lessened but they may not substitute food-related activities for drinking, when the desire for alcohol escape returns.

Since introduction of behavior modification techniques of this type has not been adequately evaluated, it is offered as a modality for trial in alcoholism rehabilitation and it will require adaptation if it is to be utilized in the various facilities provided for the care of alcoholics. In recommending staffing patterns and before making decisions on whether the health education/nutritionist should have direct responsibility for the program, or should be engaged in training the unit staff, we recommend demonstration models be established with inclusion of process and outcome evaluation procedures. Nutritionists and physicians who are interested in applying these specialized nutrition education techniques to the treatment of various categories in alcoholics in different facilities are urged to familiarize themselves with Mansell Pattison's (1974) review of rehabilitation methods for chronic alcoholics.

SELECTED REFERENCES

Anderson, M.E. 1971. Diet and the alcoholic patient. In *The Alcoholic Patient in Surgery*. Ed. Lowenfels, A.B. Baltimore: Williams and Wilkins Co. pp. 247-254.

Baker, H., Opper-Luisada, A., Sorrell, M.F., Thompson, A.D. and Frank, O. 1973. Inhibition by nicotinic acid of hepatic steatosis and alcohol dehydrogenase in ethanol-treated rats. Exper. Molec. Pathol. 19: 106-112.

Blackburn, G.L. and Bistrian, B.R. 1977. Nutritional support resources in hospital practices. In *Nutritional Support of Medical Practice*, eds. Schneider, H.A., Anderson, C.E. and Coursin, D.B. New York, San Fransisco, London: Harper and Row Publ. pp. 139-151.

Brown, D.F. 1966. The effect of ethyl α-p-chlorophenoxyisobutyrate on ethanol-induced hepatic steatosis in the rat. Metabolism 15: 868-873.

Chalmers, R.J., Sularman, W.R. and Johnson, R.H. 1977. The metabolic response to exercise in chronic alcoholics. Quart. J. Exp. Physiol. 62: 265-274.

Datsun, D.K., Santhadevi, N., Quadros, E.V., Avavi, F.C.R., Wadia, N.H., Desai, M.M. and Bharucha, E.P. 1976. The B-vitamins in malnutrition with alcoholism. A model of intervitamin relationships. Brit. J. Nutr. 36: 143-159.

Ecker, R.I. and Schroeter, A.L. 1978. Acrodermatitis and acquired zinc deficiency. Arch. Dermat. 114: 937-939.

Editorial. 1978. Dextrose, phosphorus and iron metabolism in alcoholism. Nutr. Rev. 36: 142- 144.

Faloon, W.W. 1970. Drug production of intestinal malabsorption. New York State J. Med. 70: 2189-2192.

Fenton, J.C.B., Knight, E.J. and Humpherson, P.L. 1966. Milk and cheese diet in portal-systemic encephalopathy. Lancet 1: 164-166.

Goldsmith, G.A. 1977. Curative nutrition: vitamins. In *Nutritional Support of Medical Practice*, eds. Schneider, H.A., Anderson, C.E. and Coursin, D.B. Hagerstown, MD: Harper and Row Publ. pp. 109-110.

Greenberger, N.J., Carley, J., Schenker, S., Bettinger, I., Stamnes, C. and Beyer, P. 1977. Effect of vegetable and animal protein diets in chronic hepatic encephalopathy. Amer. J. Dig. Dis. 845-855.

Hillman, R.W. 1974. Alcoholism and malnutrition. In *The Biology of Alcoholism*, Vol. 3, Clinical Pathology. Eds. Kissin, B. and Begleiter, H. New York: Plenum Press. p. 554.

Karcioglu, G.L. and Hardison, J.E. 1978. Iron-containing plasma cells. Arch. Int. Med. 138: 97-100.

Leigh Thompson, W. 19'.'8. Management of alcohol withdrawal syndromes. Arch. Intern. Med. 138: 278-283.

Lieber, C.S. 1975. Alcohol and malnutrition in the pathogenesis of liver disease. J. Amer. Med. Assoc. 233: 1077-1082.

Lieber, C.S. and DeCarli, L.M. 1970. Quantitative relationship between the amount of dietary fat and the severity of the alcoholic fatty liver. Amer. J. Clin. Nutr. 23: 474-478.

Lieber, C.S. and DeCarli, L.M. 1977. Metabolic effects of alcohol on the liver. In *Metabolic Aspects of Alcoholism,* ed. Lieber, C.S. Lancaster, England: MTP Press, Ltd. pp. 50-51.

Lieber, C.S., Lefevre, A., Spritz, N., Feinman, L. and DeCarli, L.M. 1967. Difference in hepatic metabolism of long- and medium-chain fatty acids: the role of fatty acid chain length in the production of the alcoholic fatty liver. J. Clin. Invest. 46: 1451-1460.

Lieber, C.S. and Spritz, N. 1966. Effects of prolonged ethanol intake in man: role of dietary, adipose, and endogenously synthesized fatty acids in the pathogenesis of the alcoholic fatty liver. J. Clin. Invest. 45: 1400-1411.

Maclachlan, M.J. and Rodman, G.P. 1967. Effects of food, fast and alcohol on serum uric acid and acute attacks of gout. Amer. J. Med. 42: 38-57.

Maddrey, W.C., Webber, F.L., Coulter, A.M., Chura, C.M., Chapanis, N.P. and Walser, M. 1976. Effects of keto-analogues of essential amino acids in portal-systemic encephalopathy. Gastroenterology 71: 190-195.

Mansell Pattison, E. 1974. Rehabilitation of the chronic alcoholic. In *The Biology of Alcoholism*, Vol. 3, Clinical Pathology. Eds. Kissin, B. and Begleiter, H. New York: Plenum Press. pp. 587-658.

Meng, H.C. 1977. Parenteral nutrition: Principles, nutrient requirements, techniques, and clinical application. In *Nutritional Support of Medical Practice.* Eds. Schneider, H.A., Anderson, C.E. and Coursin, D.B. Hagerstown, MD: Harper and Row Publ. pp. 152-183.

Mezey, E. 1978. Liver disease and nutrition. Gastroenterology 74: 770-783.

Mezey, E. and Potter, J.J. 1976. Changes in endocrine pancreatic function produced by altered dietary protein intake in drinking alcoholics. Johns Hopkins Med. J. 138: 7-12.

Miller, P.D., Hering, R.E. and Waterhouse, C. 1978. The treatment of alcohol acidoses: The role of dextrose and phosphorus. Arch. Intern. Med. 138: 67-72.

Ono, J., Hutson, D.G., Dombro, R.S., Levi, J.U., Livingstone, A. and Zeppa, R. 1978. Tryptophan and hepatic coma. Gastroenterology 74: 196-200.

Phear, E.A., Ruebner, B., Sherlock, S. and Summerskill, W.H.J. 1956. Methionine toxicity in liver disease and its prevention by chlortetracycline. Clin. Sci. 15: 93-117.

Richards, P. 1978. The metabolism and clinical relevance of the keto acid analogues of essential amino acids. Clin. Sci. Molec. Med. 54: 589-593.

Richards, P., Metcalfe-Gibson, A., Ward, E.E., Wrong, O.M. and Houghton, B.J. 1967. Utilization of ammonia nitrogen for protein synthesis in man, and the effect of protein restriction and anaemia. Lancet 2: 845-849.

Roe, D.A. 1976. *Drug-Induced Nutritional Deficiencies.* Westport, Conn.: AVI Publ. Co.

Roe, D.A. 1978. Physical Rehabilitation and Employment of AFDC Recipients. Final Report to the U.S.D.L., Washington, D.C.

Rudman, D., Galambos, J.T., Smith, R.B. et al. 1973. Comparison of the effect of various amino acids upon the blood ammonia concentration of patients with liver disease. Amer. J. Clin. Nutr. 26: 916-.

Rudman,D., Smith, R.B., Salam, A., Warren, W.D., Galambos, J.T. and Wegner, J. 1970. Ammonia content of food. Amer. J. Clin. Nutr. 26: 487-490.

Russell, R.M., Morrison, S.A., Rees Smith, F., Oaks, E.V. and Carney, E.A. 1978. Vitamin-A reversal of abnormal dark adaptation in cirrhosis. Study of effects on the plasma retinol transport system. Ann. Intern. Med. 88: 622-626.

Sapir, D.G. and Walser, M. 1977. Nitrogen sparing induced early in starvation by infusion of branched chain keto acids. Metabolism 26: 301-308.

Shils, M.E. 1972. Guidelines for total parenteral nutrition. J. Amer. Med. Assoc. 220: 1721-1729.

Spritz, N. and Lieber, C.S. 1966. Decrease in ethanol-induced fatty liver by ethyl α-p-chlorophenoxyisobutyrate. Proc. Soc. Exp. Biol. Med. 121: 147-149.

Thompson, G.R., Barrowman, J., Gutierrez, L., and Hermon Dowling, R. 1971. Actions of neomycin on the intraluminal phase of lipid absorption. J. Clin. Invest. 50: 319-323.

Tucker, S.B., Schroeter, A.L., Brown, P.W. Jr., and McCall, J.T. 1976. Acquired zinc deficiency. J. Amer. Med. Assoc. 235: 2399-2402.

Walser, M., Lund, P., Ruderman, N.B. and Coulter, A.W. 1973. Synthesis of essential amino acids from their alpha-keto analogues by perfused rat liver and muscle. J. Clin. Invest. 52: 2865-2877.

11

Constituents and Food Interactions of Alcohol - Containing Beverages and Drugs

NUTRITIONAL VALUE OF ALCOHOL-CONTAINING BEVERAGES, DRUGS AND INTRAVENOUS SOLUTIONS

Nutrient Composition of Alcoholic Beverages

In an account of the history of alcoholic drinks and drinking habits in Britain, Spring and Buss (1977) note that two centuries ago, intake of beer, wines and spirits provided nearly 500 kcal/person, whereas in 1975, the comparable figure was 160 kcal/person. Today, as in the past, beer has been the alcoholic beverage which contributed most in the way of nutrients as well as energy to the diet in the U.K., and most probably also in the U.S.

The energy and nutrient content of beers, wines, and liquor is shown in Table 11.1 in which values have been obtained from British and U.S. food composition tables. From this table it can be seen that beers contain B vitamins as well as essential minerals including iron, calcium, and magnesium. Wines also contain small quantities of B vitamins and minerals including iron. The iron content of certain wines and native beers, such as Kaffir beer in South Africa, are a major source of iron in the diet of heavy consumers, and may contribute to iron overload. The sodium content of alcoholic beverages is generally low, but can contribute significantly to total intake in heavy beer drinkers. Liquor contributes little to the intake of nutrients unless it is mixed with fruit juice or vegetable juice, as in the Bloody Mary cocktail.

The vitamin content of alcoholic beverages may be reduced by various factors which diminish nutrient stability, including the alcohol itself, prolonged storage, and light exposure. Photodegradation of ri-

TABLE 11.1.   ENERGY AND AVERAGE NUTRIENT CONTENT OF ALCOHOLIC BEVERAGES PER 100 ml.

Product	Energy		Na	K	Ca	Mg	P	Fe	B-vitamins*				
									Riboflavin	Niacin	B$_6$	B$_{12}$	Folacin
	Kcal	KJ	mg	mg	mg	mg	mg	mg	mg	mg	mg	µg	µg
Beer – lager	29	20	4	34	4	6	12	Tr	0.02	.33	.02	.74	4.3
Wine													
Dry White	66	275	4	61	9	8	6	0.5	0.01	.06	.02	Tr	0.2
Sweet White	94	394	14	110	14	11	13	0.58	0.01	.08	.01	Tr	0.1
Rose	71	294	4	75	12	7	6	0.95	0.01	.07	.02	Tr	0.2
Red	68	284	10	130	7	11	14	0.90**	0.02	.09	.02	Tr	0.2
Sherry-sweet	116	481	10	57	7	13	11	0.39	0.01	.10	.01	Tr	0.1
Sherry-dry	136	568	13	110	7	11	10	0.37	0.01	.07	.01	Tr	0.1
Liquor (70% proof) Average of brandy, gin, rum & whiskey	222	919	Tr	Tr	Tr	Tr	Tr	Tr	Tr	Tr	Tr	Tr	Tr

Reproduced from Paul, A.A. and Southgate, D.A.T. McCance and Widdowson's *The Composition of Foods.* Special Report No. 297, HMSO, Elsevier/North Holland Biomed Press: Amsterdam, New York, Oxford, 1978.

*B complex vitamins in beers and wines vary. Ranges given by Leake and Silverman (1971) are as follows:

	Folic Acid µg/1	Niacin µg/1	Thiamin µg/1	Riboflavin µg/1	B$_6$ µg/1	B$_{12}$ mµg/1
Beers	15-21	5000-20,000	20-60	300-1200	400-900	
Table Wines		410-960	0.240	60-220	220-820	9-25

**Iron content of wines range from <1 mg/100 ml -> 3 mg/100 ml (Davidson et al., 1975).

boflavin in beers and some wines may be minimized by use of dark bottles or cans.

The availability of micronutrients, more especially vitamins, in beer and wines may be limited by effects of ethanol on nutrient transport in the small intestine.

Since folacin deficiency is so prevalent in alcoholics, on an experimental basis, wine has been fortified with this vitamin (Kaunitz and Lindenbaum, 1977). Stability of the folic acid-fortified wine has been shown to be fairly good, though a partial loss of activity occurs with storage of the wine for two months or longer. Fortification of wine, beer and liquor with allithiamines has also been proposed (Centerwall and Criqui, 1978) as an economically beneficial method of preventing the Wernicke-Korsakoff syndrome in alcoholics. Allithiamines, which are analogues of thiamin, are better absorbed by actively drinking alcoholics than thiamin itself, and possess the same nutritional properties as the parent vitamin.

The use of wine, beer, or liquor as the vehicle for vitamins may be questioned since the imbibing public might, through a persuasive advertising campaign, be induced to believe that alcoholic beverages could not only be drunk ad libitum with impunity, but also with improvement in health. However, until such time that we are able to control alcoholism more efficiently, there is some justification for considering fortification of alcoholic beverages with stable and available vitamins as a means of preventing alcohol-related nutritional diseases, such as Korsakoff's syndrome, which leads to total disability and imposes heavy national costs for patient institutionalization.

Nutrient Content of Alcoholic Drugs

Numerous over-the-counter drugs and a much smaller number of prescription drugs contain alcohol (Bailey, 1975). Drug mixtures containing alcohol include tonics, bronchodilators and other cough medicine, cold cures, diarrhea remedies, and analgesics (Handbook of Non-Prescription Drugs, 1971). Tonics in the U.S. which contain vitamins and minerals include GeriFlex-FS (Parke Davis), and Geritol (Williams). These contain alcohol, iron and a mixture of B vitamins. Other products, such as Geroniazol (Philips, Roxane), contain alcohol and niacin. We assume that niacin is added to these products for its pharmacological effects in producing vasodilatation, rather than for nutritional advantage. The elderly may easily be persuaded to take these tonics, in order to relieve their health complaints, and perhaps to improve their memory by dilating cerebral blood vessels. While efficacy can be questioned, risk of niacin toxicity and excessive alcohol intake is limited to the abuser. Over-the-counter tonics as well as cold/cough medicines have appeal to alcoholics, both because they are an acceptable source of alcohol, and because they may contain nutrients which are believed to diminish the health risks of alcohol abuse (Table 11.2).

Ethanol in Parenteral Alimentation

Intravenous infusion of ethanol is being used in parenteral nutrition because ethanol provides a high energy source which is rapidly metabolized. It is usually administered with other nutrients including amino acid solutions. Heuckenkamp *et al.* (1976) studied effects of 5 percent ethanol-saline infusions in healthy volunteers. The ethanol was well tolerated. Urinary losses were very small and it was estimated that 98.4-98.5 percent of the ethanol was utilized. Blood glucose levels were stable within normal limits during the infusion. Blood lactate levels rose rapidly at the outset and fell when the infusion was discontinued. No hyperuricemia was observed. Effects of infusion of amino acids, sorbitol and ethanol (Aminoplex 5, Geistlich, Chester, England) on nitrogen balance in 17 patients entering a gastroenterology ward with severe nitrogen depletion were investigated by Wells and Smits (1978). Patients were divided into 3 groups: postoperative, those with inflammatory bowel disease, and those with upper gastrointestinal obstruction. The intravenous fluid was administered via a superior vena cava catheter. Intravenous vitamins (Parenterovite, Bencard, Brentford, England) were given, as well as potassium and phosphate supplements. Three different infusion rates were used. Negligible amounts of ethanol, but 9.5 percent of infused sorbitol, were excreted in the urine. Whereas plasma amino acid levels were elevated, serum urea and blood ammonia levels were not significantly elevated. As with the study in healthy patients, blood lactate levels were elevated during the infusion. As the nitrogen "intake" was increased, so urinary losses of nitrogen losses increased, particularly in patients with inflammatory bowel disease and upper GI obstruction. Restoration of nitrogen balance during the 10 day period of treatments occurred most frequently when infusion was at the highest rate. Excluding GI nitrogen losses, 14 of the 17 patients achieved positive nitrogen balance at a rate of infusion of Aminoplex 5 of 50 ml/kg/24 hrs. No metabolic complications were encountered except for moderate hypophosphatemia.

TABLE 11.2. COMMON "TONICS" AND COLD/COUGH MEDICATIONS CONTAINING ALCOHOL AND NUTRIENTS.

Product	Manufacturer	Use	Alcohol Content (%)	Nutrients Supplied	Other Active Ingredients
GeriPlex-FS	Parke Davis	Geriatric vitamin-mineral formula	18.0	Thiamin Riboflavin (FMN) Pyridoxine Vitamin B$_{12}$ Niacinamide Niacinamide Iron (ferric ammon. cit.)	Ethylene oxide + propylene oxide polymers
Geroniazol Elixir	Philips Roxane	Geriatric tonic	12.0	Niacin	Pentylene-tetrazol
Eldertonic	Mayrand	Geriatric tonic	13.5	Thiamin Riboflavin Pyridoxine Vitamin B$_{12}$ Niacinamide Folic acid Pantothenic acid (deriv.)	Caffeine
Gevrabon	Lederle	Vitamin-mineral supplement	18.0	Thiamin Riboflavin Pyridoxine Vitamin B$_{12}$ Niacinamide *Inositol *Choline *Pantothenic acid	— Minerals KI, ZnCl$_2$, MgCl$_2$, MnCl$_2$, ferrous gluconate
Geritol	Williams	Tonic	12.0	Thiamin Riboflavin Pyridoxine Niacinamide Vitamin B$_{12}$ *Panthenol (pantothenic acid) Methionine *Choline bitartrate Iron as ferric ammonium citrate	
Isuprel compound elixir	Winthrop	Expectorant Bronchodilator	19.0	Iodine as KI	Phenobarbital Isoprotarenol hydrochlor. Ephedrine Theophylline
Organidin Elixir	Wallace	Expectorant Bronchodilator	23.75	Iodine as Iodinated Glycerol	

Nutritional hazards of intravenous ethanol infusion must not be neglected. Acute folacin deficiency with pancytopenia and megaloblastic hemopoiesis has been documented by Wardrop *et al.* (1975) when Aminoplex 5 solutions were administered without adequate vitamin supplementation. The deficiency responded to folic acid. Acute folacin deficiency was conditioned by prior folacin depletion, high requirements, presence of infection and the administration of ethanol.

Ethanol as an energy source should be avoided in parenteral alimentation of alcoholics because of high risk of life-threatening folacin deficiency.

ADVERSE REACTIONS TO ALCOHOLIC BEVERAGES

Alcohol and Natural Food Toxins

1. Wild Mushrooms.—Symptoms and signs of acute food poisoning may develop when alcoholic beverages are consumed with or following a meal of wild mushrooms which are otherwise innocuous. Inky caps (*Coprinus atramentarius*) are black spored mushrooms which, when cooked and eaten, produce no adverse effects except when alcohol is taken. The combination of *C. atramentarius* and alcohol produces an acetaldehyde-like reaction which is similar to, or identical with, that produced by disulfiram (Antabuse) (Buck, 1961).

Simandl and Franc (1956) claimed isolation of disulfiram from *C. atramentarius*, but subsequent investigations, discussed by Tyler (1963), did not confirm this finding. Symptoms that follow intake of alcohol with *C. atramentarius* include flushing, palpitations, dyspnea, hyperventilation, sometimes transient hypertension, tachycardia, nausea, vomiting, and collapse. The severity of the reaction is dependent both on the amount of alcoholic beverage consumed and on the amount of *C. atramentarius* eaten. Symptoms usually last for about two hours, and then subside.

Temporal relationships between the intake of these mushrooms and the alcohol, as well as the method of preparation of the mushrooms, may influence the appearance or nonappearance of the reaction. In some instances, alcoholic beverages can be taken immediately after the mushrooms, but a reaction occurs if the alcohol is consumed several hours and at least up to 24 hours later. However, other people do react if they drink alcohol before or during the time that the mushrooms are eaten. If the mushrooms are eaten raw, it is reported that they do not induce the reaction. Smith (1958), when he described the characteristics and culinary use of Inky Cap mushrooms, only mentioned the alcohol reactions as occurring with *C. atramentarius* and not with other members of that mushroom family. This specific toxic effect of *C. atramentarius* is also mentioned by Sapeika (1969).

Reynolds and Lowe (1963) described 4 people, 2 men and 2 women, who ate several different species of mushroom including Inky Caps and 24 hours later beer was drunk by 3 of the 4 people. Within minutes of drinking the beer, the typical reaction occurred. However, one individual drank beer within 3 hours of the mushroom meal and had only mild tingling of the hands and feet. Others in the party who had eaten the mushrooms at a common meal, but without drinking beer later on, had no ill effects. There was no history of disulfiram ingestion by any of these 4 patients.

2. Fish.—Fish poisoning which is variously known as Ciguatera poisoning, Ichthyosarcotoxism, or Gymnothrax poisoning, occurs under special circumstances when fish from certain waters (e.g. in the Caribbean and Pacific areas) is eaten. The poison is not peculiar to any one fish, but is acquired via the food chain many species including groupers, sea bass, parrot fish, eels, barracuda, mackeral, surgeon fish, snapper, jacks, perch, and any other fish which live on blue-green algae. The Ciguatera toxin is contained mainly in the liver and viscera of the fish, but may be also present in the fish skin and muscle. Onset of symptoms is within 36 hours of ingestion of the fish. Symptoms include paresthesias such as itching and intense burning of the skin, as well as neurological symptoms including blurring of vision, ataxia and convulsions, and gastrointestinal symptoms including nausea and vomiting. In severe cases of poisoning by this fish toxin, convulsions and motor paralysis may develop. Through personal observation by the author, it is seen that when alcoholic beverages including beer, wine, and liquor are consumed, even in very small amounts after the appearance of Ciguatera poisoning, intense itching of the skin occurs within 15-30 min. and lasts 2-3 hours or longer. This peculiar effect of alcohol on Ciguatera food poisoning induced by alcohol may persist for about 10 days (Sapeika, 1969; Schantz, 1973; Moffie and Haneveld, 1964; Russell, 1971; Roe, personal observation).

MONAMINE OXIDASE INHIBITOR DRUGS, WINE, AND HYPERTENSION

Monamine oxidase inhibitor drugs (MAOI) all block oxidative deamination of endogenous and exogenous amines such as tyramine and dopamine which are present in certain foods and wine. Structurally dissimilar drugs, sharing the MAOI property, have been used for their mood elevating effect in neurotic and psychotic depression. These drugs form complexes with monamine oxidase and inhibit its metabolic degradation.

Since publication of a report by Asatoor (1963), hypertensive crises have been recognized as the most serious side effect of MAOI drugs. These crises follow intake of certain foods including cheese, yeast or yeast extract (Marmite), chicken liver, broad beans, pickled herring, as well as beer and wine, by patients receiving MAOI inhibitors (Thomas, 1963; Sapeika, 1969). Symptoms appear 30-60 min. after the offending food or beverage is consumed. Complaints are of headache, palpitations, nausea, and vomiting. Transient but often severe hypertensive attacks occur, and cerebral hemorrhage is reported as the cause of death in fatal cases.

Attacks vary in occurrence and severity with the specific MAOI drug dosage level and the intake of tyramine. Certain wines, notably Chianti, have a high tyramine content. Hepatic tyramine metabolism is inhibited by MAOI drugs. Non-metabolized tyramine releases norepinephrine from nerve endings, where it is believed that this catacholamine is present in higher than normal concentrations in patients receiving these drugs.

Prescribing of MAOI drugs as antidepressants has been limited since the risk of hypertensive attacks has been recognized. Drugs in the group presently available in the U.S. are: Isocarboxazide, Nialamid, Phenelzine, and Tranylcypromine. Tyrer et al. (1973) have advocated use of MAOI drugs in the treatment of phobic anxiety and in combination with the tricyclic antidepressants, Amitriptline or Trimipramine, in "refractory" depressive illnesses.

Alcoholics are at risk for hypertensive side effects of these drugs, a) because they are likely to be over-represented in groups of depressed patients, and are likely to have refractory depression; b) because they may consume large quantities of wine containing tyramine; and c) because they are unlikely to remember to refrain from eating cheeses and other high tyramine foods when given MAOI antidepressants.

Procarbazine, a drug of choice in the treatment of Hodgkins disease, is a weak MAOI drug. Hypertension has been described in patients eating tyramine-containing foods or drinking tyramine-containing beverages while on Procarbazine therapy (Spivack, 1974).

A list of tyramine-containing foods and beverages is given in Table 11.3 with actual figures for tyramine content.

TABLE 11.3   TYRAMINE CONTENT OF ALCOHOLICS' BEVERAGES AND FOODS.

Product	Tyramine ($\mu g/g$ or $\mu g/ml$)
Wines:	
Chianti	25.4
Sherry	3.6
Sauterne	0.4
Riesling	0.6
Cheeses:	
New York State Cheddar	1416.0
Stilton	466.0
Gruyere	516.0
Processed American	50.0

Taken from Horwitz, D., W. Lovenberg, K. Engelman and A. Sjoerdsma. J. Amer. Med. Assoc. 188: 90-94, 1964.

THE DISULFIRAM REACTION AND RELATED ALCOHOL-DRUG EFFECTS

Tetraethylthiuram disulfide (disulfiram/Antabuse) is used extensively in the management of alcoholics in order to force abstinence. If alcohol is drunk when the alcoholic patient is receiving this drug, disagreeable symptoms occur within 5-15 min. Flushing of the face, neck and upper chest and occasionally the arms is followed or sometimes accompanied by a throbbing headache. Nausea follows, and is variable in degree and in the time at which it is experienced after ingestion of alcohol. Morgan and Cagan (1974) observed that nausea will begin 30-60 min. after taking 40-50 g alcohol. According to these authors, disulfiram has two effects: it increases blood and tissue acetaldehyde levels, and it also causes depletion of norepinephrine in many tissues including the brain, heart, and adrenal glands. They speculate that perhaps the increase in acetaldehyde level causes the norepinephrine depletion secondarily. With the development of nausea the patient becomes pale and may feel faint. A fall in blood pressure may occur, but is by no means a uniform effect. Vague, unlocalized, abdominal pain and vomiting may follow the development of nausea. Patients feel uneasy or actually frightened. Hyperventilation is common. Chest pain, which may be unilateral and usually left-sided, as well as vertigo and blurred vision, may bring the patient to his doctor's office, or to the accident room of the local hospital. Psychotic reactions may be induced by disulfiram, particularly in patients who have previously been schizophrenic.

Alcoholics receiving disulfiram will develop the typical alcohol-related reaction not only when they drink alcoholic beverages, but also when they eat foods containing liquor, wine or beer. The severity of the reaction is related not only to the amount of alcohol taken, but also to the dose of the drug received.

Disulfiram-like reaction occurs with ingestion of alcoholic beverages or consumption of foods containing alcohol with any of the following drugs: furazolidone, griseofulvin, quinacrine, metronidazole, procarbazine, tolazoline, chlorpropamide. With some of these drugs the reaction may be brought about by inhibition of aldehyde dehydrogenase (Griffin and D'Arcy, 1975).

Citrated calcium carbimide, which has been used in Canada and Japan as a substitute for disulfiram, produces identical side effects (Seixas, 1975).

The anthelmintic, tetrachlorethylene, produces a peculiar susceptibility to ethanol such that reactions have some of the characteristics of the disulfiram reaction. In particular, if alcohol is taken when patients are receiving the drug, or alcohol is consumed by workers who are manufacturing tetrachlorethylene, then profound flushing of the skin occurs. Sedation occurs also, through the additive effects of alcohol and tetrachlorethylene, when these two drugs are taken together.

ALLERGIC REACTIONS TO CHEMICAL ADDITIVES IN ALCOHOLIC DRINKS

Allergic reactions may occur following ingestion of or contact with alcoholic beverages containing food chemicals. Contact dermatitis may be due to flavoring agents used in liqueurs, aperitifs and mixers. The common food flavoring agents which cause contact dermatitis are anise seed oil, almond oil, benzaldehyde, capsicum, carroway oil, cinnamon oil, ginger oil, limonene oil, menthol and peppermint oil. Reactivation of contact dermatitis will occur when drinks are taken containing these agents. Bartenders as well as alcoholics are particularly at risk (Adams, 1969).

Allergic purpura may occur in drinkers who take gin and tonic or drinks containing Campari, due to quinine sensitivity. Another source of quinine which can give rise to purpura is the drink Bitter Lemon, which may be used as a mixer. Quinine cannot only cause allergic purpura, but also thrombocytopenic purpura. Urticaria in drinkers may be due to tartrazine, which is a coloring agent in sodas and other soft drinks used as mixers, to salicylates or menthol present in gums and candy used as a breath deodorant, or due to any one of the flavoring agents which were cited as causes of contact dermatitis. Vasodilitation induced by alcohol consumption may exacerbate the itching due to urticaria. A fixed drug eruption has been reported from use of disulfiram. Disappearance of the fixed drug eruptions would indicate that the drug was not being taken as prescribed because it is the characteristic of this dermatosis to develop and reappear in the same sites with drug intake (Beerman *et al.*, 1967).

ACUTE HYPOGLYCEMIA

Acute hypoglycemia may develop in those who take mixed alcoholic drinks on an empty stomach. Under these circumstances, the combined effects of alcohol and sugar cause reactive hypoglycemia and associated symptoms. O'Keefe and Marx (1977) studied ten young subjects who drank either 3 gin and tonics containing 50 g alcohol and 60 g sucrose, gin with a low calorie tonic containing 0.5 g sucrose, or a tonic water alone, containing 60 g sucrose. Behavior of the subjects, their symptoms, their blood glucose and plasma insulin levels were monitored subsequently for 5 hours. Both alcohol-containing drinks caused mild inebriation; only the gin with regular tonic water containing a substantial amount of sugar had a significant effect on glucose and plasma insulin. Peak insulin levels were higher when regular gin and tonic was taken than when the mixed drink contained gin and the low sugar mixer. In three subjects, behavioral changes suggestive of hypoglycemia were present during the period when blood sugar levels were lowest, following the regular gin and tonic routine.

The authors emphasized that their experiment mimics the common situation when alcohol with a sugar mixer is taken in the fasting state. Results indicate that it is the combination of sucrose and alcohol which gives rise to a more severe reactive hypoglycemia and that this combination can result in behavioral changes appearing. Alcohol alone can cause hyperinsulinemia, probably because of a direct effect on the beta cells of the pancreas. The investigators in the gin and tonic experiment believe that alcohol may cause release of an intestinal polypeptide, affecting insulin release, when hyperglycemia is present. In other words, they consider that the reactive hypoglycemia which they found in their subjects was due to a combined and perhaps synergistic effect of alcohol and sugar on insulin secretion.

Alcohol enhances the hypoglycemia effects of sulfonyl urea drugs, used as antidiabetic agents. These drugs which are used in the management of maturity-onset diabetes, stimulate pancreatic islet tissue to secrete insulin (Larner and Haynes, 1975; Editorial, JAMA, 1968; Moss, 1969).

HANGOVER EFFECTS - A MATTER OF CONGENERS?

Scientific and lay experience suggests that hangover effects after drinking are worse following consumption of distilled beverages of high rather than low congener content. Congeners are pharmacologically active molecules, other than ethanol, present in alcoholic beverages including acetaldehyde, ethyl formate, ethyl acetate, methanol, n-propanol, n-butanol, and iso-amyl alcohol. Three of the higher alcohols, n-propyl, n-butyl, and iso-amyl alcohol, are the most abundant of these byproducts in liquors. Examples of liquors of high congener content include bourbon whiskey, rum and brandy, whereas vodka has a low congener content (Table 11.4). Murphree and Price (1966), Murphree et al. (1967), and Murphree (1969) showed that whereas both bourbon and vodka had effects on quantitative electroencephalograms, simulating those produced by tranquilizers, bourbon induced a greater incidence of EEG effects. Further, drowsiness was greater with bourbon than with vodka.

TABLE 11.4.   CONGENER CONTENTS OF SYNTHETIC ETHANOL, VODKA, AND BOURBON (mg/100 ml)

	Ethanol	Vodka	Bourbon
Acetaldehyde	0.3	0.3	1.7
Ethyl formate	0.8	0.4	2.7
Ethyl acetate	0.0	0.0	82.5
Methanol	0.5	0.4	2.6
n-Propanol	0.0	0.0	11.0
i-Butanol	0.0	0.0	25.0
i-Amyl alcohol	0.0	0.0	120.0

Taken from Sardesai, V.M., ed. Biochemical and Clinical Aspects of Alcohol Metabolism. Springfield, IL: Charles C. Thomas, 1969, p. 260.

Kissin (1974) has indicated that whereas interaction between ethanol and congeners in alcoholic beverages may explain the hangover effect, studies to date are suggestive but not conclusive.

Indeed, when Auty and Branch (1978) administered ethanol alone, ethanol plus a mixture of higher alcohols (n-propanol, n-butanol, and isoamyl alcohol) or whiskey to normal volunteers at a dose equivalent to 1 g/kg body weight, plasma ethanol concentration profiles following the test were similar. The time to reach peak plasma concentration of ethanol was greater with whiskey than with the other beverages though the area under the plasma concentration time curves was similar. Deterioration in performance, 2 hours after ingestion, was less with whiskey than with the other beverages. EEG changes were not significantly different between treatment groups. Subjects were unable to distinguish between beverages which were diluted with orange juice. No evidence was obtained to suggest that whiskey had any different effect than ethanol. It is to be pointed out however, that all beverages were highly diluted (up to 600 ml) at the time of administration which could have influenced outcome. Subjective evidence of hangovers was not investigated.

Non-alcoholic male volunteers studied by Pawan (1973) were given red wine, white wine, rum, whiskey, gin, vodka, brandy, and diluted pure ethanol (20 percent) in orange juice. The amount of each drink consumed was 1.5 ml ethanol/kg body weight. Symptoms reported thereafter were headache, tiredness, nausea, and other GI disturbances. Hangover effects were related to the congener content of the drinks, and were produced most frequently by brandy, followed by red wine, rum, whiskey, white wine and gin, in that order. Vodka and diluted ethanol produced the least hangover effects.

Ylikahri et al. (1974) demonstrated that the severity of hangover shows interindividual variability and is related to the degree of metabolic acidosis. Induction of metabolic acidosis is not known to be related to specific congener content of alcoholic beverages. We therefore need to study whether any one, or any group, of non-ethanolic components of these beverages is more liable than others to produce metabolic acidosis, to learn whether variability in hangover effects is related to rates of congener metabolism and whether the sugar or ascorbic acid content of orange juice protects against congener toxicity.

SELECTED REFERENCES

Adams, R.M. 1969. *Occupational Contact Dermatitis.* Philadelphia, Toronto: J.B. Lippincott Co. pp. 93, 238.

Asatoor, A.M., Levi, A.J. and Milne, M.D. 1963. Tranlcypromine and cheese. Lancet 2: 733-734.

Auty, R.M. and Branch, R.A. 1978. Pharmacokinetics and pharmacodynamics of ethanol, whiskey and ethanol with n-propyl, n-butyl and iso-amyl alchols. Clin. Pharm. Therap. 22: 242-248.

Bailey, D. 1975. The alcohol content of some commonly prescribed medicines. J. Alcoholism 10: 67-72.

Beerman, H., Kirshbaum, B.A. and Criep, L.H. 1967. Adverse drug reactions. In *Dermatologic Allergy: Immunology, Diagnosis, Management.* Philadelphia and London: W.B. Saunders Co. pp. 189-221.

Buck, R.W. 1961. Mushroom toxins - brief review of literature. New Eng. J. Med. 265: 681-686.

Centerwall, B.S. and Criqui, M.H. 1978. Prevention of the Wernicke-Korsakoff syndrome. A cost-benefit analysis. New Eng. J. Med. 299: 285-289.

Davidson, S., Passmore, R., Brock, J.F. and Truswell, A.S. 1975. *Human Nutrition and Dietetics.* 6th ed. Edinburgh, London, New York: Churchill Livingston.

Editorial. 1968. Alcohol and hypoglycemia coma. J. Amer. Med. Assoc. 206: 639-642.

Griffin, J.P. and D'Arcy, P.F. 1975. *A Manual of Adverse Drug Reaction.* Bristol, England: John Wright & Sons, Ltd. pp. 60-61.

Handbook of Non-Prescription Drugs. 1971. Eds. Griffenhagen, B.G. and Hawkins, L.L. Amer. Pharmaceut. Assoc., Washington, D.C.

Heuckenkamp, P-U., Sprandel, U. and Liebhardt, E.W. 1977. Studies concerning ethanol as a nutrient for intravenous alimentation in man. Nutr. Metab. 21, Suppl. 1: 121-124.

Kanuitz, J.D. and Lindenbaum, J. 1977. The bioavailability of folic acid added to wine. Ann. Intern. Med. 87: 542-545.

Larner, J. and Haynes, R.C. 1975. Insulin and oral hypoglycemic drugs: Glucagon. In *The Pharmacological Basis of Therapeutics.* Eds. Goodman, L.S. and Gilman, A. 5th ed., New York: Macmillan Co. pp. 1519-1523.

Leake, C.D. and Silverman, M. 1971. The chemistry of alcoholic beverages. In *The Biology of Alcoholism,* Vol. 1, Biochemistry. Eds. Kissin, B. and Begleiter, H. New York and London: Plenum Press. pp. 575-612.

Moffie, D. and Haneveld, G.T. 1964. Ciguatera fish poisoning in the Caribbean area. Nederl. T. Geneesk. 108: 88-.

Morgan, R. and Cagan, E.J. 1974. Acute alcohol intoxication, the disulfiram reaction and methylalcohol intoxication. In *The Biology of Alcoholism,* Vol. 3. Eds. Kissin, B. and Begleiter, H. New York and London: Plenum Press. pp. 163-189.

Moss, J.M. 1969. Cocktails and diabetes. Gen. Prac. 40: 129-.

Murphree, H.B. 1969. Effects of alcoholic beverages containing large and small amounts of congeners. In *Biochemical and Clinical Aspects of Alcohol Metabolism.* Ed. Sardesai, V.M. Springfield, Il: Charles C. Thomas. pp. 259-265.

Murphree, H.B., Greenberg, L.A. and Carroll, R.B. 1967. Neuropharmacoligical effects of substances other than ethanol in alcoholic beverages. Fed. Proc. 26: 1468-1473.

Murphree, H.B. and Price, L.M. 1966. Computer time - series analysis of the EEG effects of alcoholic beverages. Fed. Proc. 25: 503-511.

O'Keefe, S.J.D. and Marx, V. 1977. Lunch-time gin and tonic. A cause of reactive hypoglycaemia. Lancet 1: 1286-1287.

Pawan, G.L.S. 1973. Alcoholic drinks and hangover effects. Proc. Nutr. Soc. 32: 15A.

Reynolds, W.A. and Lowe, S.H. 1965. Mushrooms and a toxic reation to alcohol. Report of 4 cases. New Eng. J. Med. 272: 630-631.

Russell, F.E. 1971. Pharmacology of toxins of marine organisms. In *International Encyclopedia of Pharmacology and Therapeutics.* Sec. 71: Pharmacology and Toxicology of Naturally Occurring Toxins. Vol. 2. Oxford. New York, Toronto, Sidney: Pergamon Press. pp.3-114.

Sapieka, N. 1969. *Food Pharmacology.* Springfield, Il: Charles C. Thomas Co. pp. 54, 93-94, 104.

Schantz, E.J. 1973. Seafood toxicants. In *Toxicants Occurring Naturally in Foods,* 2nd ed. NAS, Washington, D.C. pp. 424-447.

Seixas, F.A. 1975. Alcohol and its drug interactions. Ann. Intern. Med. 83: 86-92.

Simandl, J. and Franc, J. 1956. Isolation of tetraethylthiuram disulfide from *Coprinus atramentarius.* Chem. Listy. 50: 1862-1869.

Smith, A.H. 1958. *The Mushroom Hunters Field Guide.* AnnArbor, Michigan: Univ. Michigan Press. pp. 153-158.

Spivak, S.D. 1974. Procarbazine. Ann. Intern. Med. 81: 795-800.

Spring, J.A. and Buss, D.H. 1977. Three centuries of alcohol in the British diet. Nature 270: 567-572.

Thomas, J.C.S. 1963. Monamine oxidase inhibitors in cheese. Brit. Med. J. 2: 1406-1410.

Tyler, V.E., Jr. 1963. Poisonous mushrooms. Progr. in Chem. Toxicol. 1: 339-384.

Tyrer, P., Candy, J. and Kelly, D. 1973. A study of the clinical effects of phenelzine and placebo in the treatment of phobic anxiety. Psychopharmacologia 32: 237-254.

Wardrop, C.A.J., Tennant, G.B., Heatley, R.V. and Hughes, L.E. 1975. Acute folate deficiency in surgical patients on amino acid/ethanol intravenous nutrition. Lancet 2: 640-642.

Wells, F.E. and Smits, B.J. 1978. Utilization and metabolic effects of a solution of amino acids, sorbitol and ethanol in parenteral nutrition. Amer. J. Clin. Nutr. 31: 442-450.

Ylikahri, R.H., Poso, A.R., Huhunen, M.O. and Hilborn, M.E. 1974. Alcohol intoxication and hangover. Effects on plasma electrolyte concentrations and acid-base balance. Scand. J. Clin. Lab. Invest. 34: 327-336.

Index

Other AVI Books